Drugs During Pregnancy
Clinical Perspectives

TO
MY PARENTS,
WADI' AND ALICE

Drugs During Pregnancy
Clinical Perspectives

RAJA W. ABDUL-KARIM, M.D.
Professor, Department of Obstetrics and Gynecology
State University of New York
Upstate Medical Center
Syracuse, New York

With Contributions By

HOWARD J. OSOFSKY, M.D., PH.D.
Staff and Research Psychiatrist, The Menninger Foundation, Clinical
Professor of Obstetrics and Gynecology, University of Kansas Medical
Center

DONALD R. MATTISON, M.D.
Pregnancy Research Branch, National Institutes of Child Health,
Bethesda, MD.

ROGER SCOTT, J.D.
Attorney and Partner, Scott, Sardano and Pomeranz, Syracuse, New York

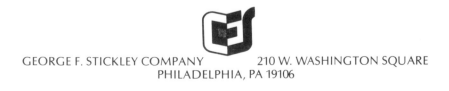

GEORGE F. STICKLEY COMPANY   210 W. WASHINGTON SQUARE
PHILADELPHIA, PA 19106

Printed and Manufactured in the United States and published by the George F. Stickley Company, 210 West Washington Square, Phila., Pa. 19106.

Contents

(continued on next page)

CONTENTS (continued)

FOREWORD

"In nature's infinite book of secrecy
A little I can read." *Shakespeare*

The realization that substances ingested during pregnancy could harm the unborn was acknowledged in ancient times. (Newlyweds in Sparta were cautioned against alcohol intake.) However, it was only in the early 1960's, after what has come to be known as the "thalidomide tragedy," that the current widespread concern among physicians and their patients arose over the potential harmful effects of drugs taken during pregnancy.

It is a truism of sound medical practice that unnecessary drugs should not be taken during pregnancy (and one may add, by the nonpregnant as well). The fact remains, however, that not infrequently the need for medications will occur during pregnancy and, in addition to other considerations, raises the issue of potential effects on the fetus. Herein lies the crux of the problem, for the precise knowledge needed about the fetal effect of drugs is more often lacking than available.

This is primarily due to the unavailability of the required studies in humans, for in the last analysis, potential human fetal effects can only be ascertained by observations in the human. This book, which is not intended to be an all-inclusive catalogue for drugs and pregnancy, was written with the above considerations in mind. Its purpose is to bring into proper perspective many of the special issues involved with the use of drugs during pregnancy and their effects on the fetus.

I am indebted to Dr. Donald Mattison for providing the chapter on "The Effects of Biologically Foreign Compounds on Reproduction," to Dr. Howard Osofsky for the section on "Psychotropic Drugs," and to Dr. Thelma Yambao for her contribution to the section on "Antibiotics."

The invaluable help rendered by my research assistant, Mary Haviland, and my secretary, Suzanne LaManna, in preparing the manuscript is gratefully acknowledged. I am also grateful for the assistance, cooperation, and understanding of Margot Newman Stickley and George F. Stickley of the George F. Stickley Company.

Raja W. Abdul-Karim, M.D.

DRUGS IN PREGNANCY— AN OVERVIEW

"For true understanding, comprehension of detail is imperative. Since such detail is well-nigh infinite, our knowledge is always superficial and imperfect." *de La Rochefoucauld*

The problem facing the clinician utilizing drugs in pregnancy is that despite widespread interest and vigilance, very few drugs are accepted as being definitely teratogenic in man; and even among these few, some disagreement is present. Those drugs considered definitely teratogenic in man include thalidomide, folic acid antagonists, and androgenic hormones. Other drugs that could fall into this category are antithyroid medications, tetracyclines and diethylstilbestrol. Thalidomide, an "ideal" human teratogen, produces a fairly well defined pattern of anomalies, mainly of limb and face. Androgenic hormones including synthetic progestogen cause masculinization of the genitalia in female fetuses. Folic acid antagonists and alkylating agents have a devastating effect on the conceptus; there is a high rate of embryonic or fetal death and a high incidence of congenital anomalies in those that survive. The latter is more clearly documented in the folic acid antagonists, due partly to the paucity of experience and the high rate of intrauterine death with alkylating agents. Diethylstilbestrol (DES) causes abnormalities in the histogenesis of the vaginal epithelium and other abnormalities in both the male and female genital tracts. Thyroid suppressants, e.g., thiourea, may cause congenital goiter.

It is of some comfort to realize that drugs such as DES, thalidomide, and androgenic compounds have no known therapeutic value during pregnancy; hence, future concern about their fetal effects should not arise. However, the need for anticancer drugs, though infrequent, will regrettably arise. Here the option for therapeutic abortion is present. Consequently, fetal anomalies due to drugs of established teratogenicity should not become a pressing problem in clinical practice. The problem resides in the multitude of other drugs that may become needed during pregnancy, where the teratogenic potential in the human is unknown or largely a matter of debate.

PERSPECTIVES ON THE TERATOGENICITY OF DRUGS

The difficulties encountered in assessing the impact of environmental factors in general on human teratology apply equally well to the more specific issue of drugs and pregnancy outcome. Despite the likelihood of an increase in exposure to possible teratogens, and the heightened overall alertness to the problem, the overall incidence of congenital malformations does not appear on the rise. Specific examples of a sudden increase in congenital defects have occurred, but here the cause is almost always readily identifiable since it exhibits a strong teratogenic influence. Thalidomide is a clear example in which a specific teratogen was identified, and with its removal a demonstrable decrease in anomalies occurred. Such examples are rare, however.

The view may be expressed that the lack of an obvious overall increase in congenital anomalies argues against an increase in exposure to teratogenic influences. Such an approach is ill advised for, if nothing else, it would serve to lower our vigilance. There are other more plausible explanations. The anomalous zygotes, embryos, or fetuses may either be spontaneously or willfully aborted. The prevalence of these abnormalities is almost impossible to determine since such products of gestation are not always available or amenable to critical examination. On the other hand, it may be too soon to assess the outcome, especially when minor and/or functional abnormalities are considered. The evaluation of changes in potential functional aptitudes is a most difficult and exacting task. This leads us into the issue of statistical power.

An agent that is strongly teratogenic reveals itself rather quickly and—if the pregnancy reaches beyond the period of viability—could leave in its wake a significant number of abnormal offspring. A weak teratogen, on the other hand, can escape detection for long periods of time, because a large population is needed to show 1) that the incidence of the observed effect has in fact changed, and 2) that the change was due to the agent in question. For example, if the incidence of an anomaly is 1:1000 in unexposed pregnancies and 2:1000 in exposed pregnancies, it would take over 20,000 subjects to detect this difference with an acceptable power at conventional test levels. These numbers are not easy to attain. They are important, however, in order to avoid the errors of insufficient sampling. Smaller numbers may not show a significant effect, not because the effect is not there, but because the sample was inadequate to achieve a statistical significance; or the opposite may occur.

The incidence of malformations shows seasonal, geographic and socioeconomic associations. It also varies with parental age and sex of the offspring. The cause of the former is largely unknown. There is no clear explanation for the varying geographical incidence of cleft palate or anencephaly. The apparent decrease in Down's syndrome in some communities may be due to the changing maternal age. Studies on teratology should consider all of these factors in their analysis.

INCIDENCE OF DRUG USE DURING PREGNANCY

An overwhelming majority of women ingest one or more drugs during their pregnancy. If vitamins and minerals are included, the figure is close to 100%. This large intake of drugs is not limited to vitamins and minerals but includes among others, antibiotics, antacids, analgesics, antiemetics, antidepressants, antihistamines, diuretics, hypnotics, narcotics, appetite suppressants, hormones—not to mention illicit drugs, alcohol, caffeine, and the many other chemical agents found in various foods and drinks.

In a survey by Forfar and Nelson (1973) of drugs used in pregnancy (excluding iron) 82% of the women were taking prescribed drugs; 65% took self-prescribed drugs. Excluding iron and vitamins, the medications included antidepressants and sedatives (32%), antibiotics (28%), diuretics (18%), antiemetics (16%), analgesics (15%), antacids (11%). Another report showed that 32% of the subjects took diuretics, 17% antihistamines, 24% analgesics, 14% appetite suppressants, and 14% hypnotics and narcotics. Twenty-one percent of the women received more than five drugs, and about 4% ten or more (Peckham and King, 1963).

Hill and co-workers (1977) interviewed 231 pregnant women between 1969-1975 regarding drugs taken during pregnancy: 0-37 preparations were recorded with a mean of 15.6. The range for prescribed drugs was 0-28 with a mean of 6.4 per patient. Over-the-counter drugs averaged 3.2 drugs per patient (range 0-12). Ninety-five percent of the women took one or more "over-the-counter drugs." In a small number of patients the nature of the drug consumed could not be identified.

Doering and Stewart (1978) reported medication consumption in 168 pregnant women. Over 90% of these patients ingested five or more medications; the average number of drug products taken was 11 per subject. Since many of the drug products consumed contained more than one ingredient, the total number of chemicals to which both mother and fetus were exposed would be higher. In the table classifying drug consumption per therapeutic category, the authors listed 44 (26.2%) patients under "unknown medications." Thus it is apparent that a large number of drugs are consumed by pregnant women and that not all of the medications taken are prescribed by a physician. Many are "over-the-counter drugs" that the patient obtains without a prescription. Consequently, the physician may not even be aware of all of the medications his patient has received, either through lack of reporting or inability to trace the nature of the preparation. Notwithstanding such observations, the majority of drugs taken during pregnancy appear to be prescribed.

Indeed, vitamins and iron apart, it seems that pregnant women tend to receive more prescriptions for drugs than a matched group of non-pregnant controls. This may be explained by the increased predilection of pregnant women to such disorders as nausea, vomiting, heartburn, various aches and pains, phlebothrombosis, and possibly, anxiety and insomnia.

DIFFICULTIES IN ASSESSING
DRUG TERATOGENICITY IN THE HUMAN

Not infrequently, drugs (self- or physician-prescribed) are taken before it is realized that conception has occurred. This possibility should be entertained in all fertile women, and a careful menstrual history obtained. Special considerations should be given to medications in the latter half of a menstrual cycle since here the potential for pregnancy exists. Furthermore, patients may not consider the possibility that non-prescription medications could be harmful to the fetus. Consequently, patient education to the potential harmful effects of all drugs on the fetus is an important responsibility of the physician.

There are other problems associated with drug intake during

pregnancy and its effects on the fetus. There is as yet no experimental animal that can in all aspects substitute for the human./ This fact was forcefully underscored by the thalidomide tragedy. Thalidomide, a relatively innocuous drug to some animals is a powerful teratogen in the human. This high degree of teratogenicity was not apparent in many of the animal species on which the drug was tested. The reverse may also sometimes be true. It follows, therefore, that extrapolation to the human of the results of animal testing is not always a reliable phenomenon and caution is to be exercised. In the last analysis, the question of drug teratogenicity in the human can only be completely answered by human observations. These, as will be discussed further in more detail, are not easy to obtain. Some of the factors adding to the difficulties include: the paucity of knowledge on drug metabolism in—and how it may be modified by—pregnancy (studies on drug metabolism in the human are almost universally carried out on non-pregnant subjects; drug distribution, binding and elimination may be altered by the hypoalbuminemia, increased total body water, and increased renal clearance associated with pregnancy); the inability to discern the effect of the drug from that of the concurrent disease; the multiplicity of drugs ingested, hence the difficulty in identifying the effect of a single from that of a group of drugs and/or drug interactions; the inability to differentiate the effect of drugs from that of their metabolites or from the many chemical and other environmental factors a pregnant woman is exposed to; and finally, the adverse effect of a drug on the fetus which may become apparent only after birth and which may not be demonstrable as an obvious morphologic or structural abnormality.

For obvious reasons it is difficult to carry out well-controlled studies on teratogens in the human. In addition, it is not feasible with present techniques to properly assess the pharmacology of a drug in the mother and her fetus, the transfer of the drug to the fetus and its placental metabolism, and the influence of gestational age. Most studies relating to these matters are done near or at term and principally involve comparisons of maternal and fetal blood levels. Similar approaches have been carried out at the time of induced abortion, but here again the emphasis is mainly on blood levels, and to a lesser extent on distribution and metabolism. With these techniques, effects on morphogenesis, or function remain unknown. Direct studies to assess these aspects fully are, to our knowledge, unknown in the human. This knowledge, then, is primarily derived from epidemiologic analysis, with its necessary drawbacks.

In the last analysis, the evaluation of drug teratogenicity in the human can only be derived by administering the drug to humans and studying its effects. In prescribing drugs during pregnancy the physician is frequently acting in an area where insufficient clinical knowledge and incomplete and contradictory data exist. This may produce a great deal of anxiety and hesitancy in prescribing drugs for the pregnant female. To the extent that this hesitancy results in a careful and balanced assessment of the need for such medication—with careful consideration of possible alternatives, side effects, etc.—it is deserved and well-served. If this practice, however, leads to denying a pregnant woman an indicated medication for her particular illness, the practice is ill-advised. Not only is the mother's health and welfare jeopardized, but so is that of her unborn child. No woman should be denied *needed* drugs for fear of real or potential fetal harm. The drug of comparable efficacy and least harm should be used when a choice is available. The patient should be made aware of all known aspects in regard to indications, benefits, and risks. She may elect to accept or refuse. In the last analysis, it is the well-informed patient who makes the choice.

ASSESSMENT OF DRUG EFFECTS ON REPRODUCTION

The "thalidomide tragedy" in the early '60s represents the pivotal point that led to stricter and more comprehensive guidelines for testing drug effects on reproduction. Prior to this event, recommendations concerning the evaluation of drug effects on reproduction revolved around conventional chronic toxicity tests. In 1966 the Food and Drug Administration issued its "Guidelines for Reproduction Studies for Safety Evaluation of Drugs for Human Use"; and subsequently, protocols on additives and pesticide residues were formulated (Toxicol. Appl. Pharmacol. 16:264, 1970). Other countries have introduced comparable requirements. Although not faultless, these guidelines represent a major development toward the perceived goal.

A general outline delineating the scope of the requirements for drug testing on reproduction is provided in the following table. Specific recommendations and requirements vary among countries.

Recently the Food and Drug Administration (FDA Drug Bulletin, DHEW: Pregnancy Labeling, 9:23, 1979) instituted five categories to describe the teratogenic potential of drugs. This infor-

TABLE 1. REQUIREMENTS OF DRUG TESTING ON REPRODUCTION

1. Animals (males and females) treated *before* mating and throughout pregnancy for effects on:
   A. Gametogenesis
   B. Fertility
   C. Fetus at various gestational ages (e.g., mutations, abortions, fetal death, anomalies, etc.)
2. Animals treated during critical period, latter part of pregnancy or throughout pregnancy. Effect of drug and/or metabolites on:
   A. Fetal and uterine growth
   B. Embryotoxicity-congenital malformations
   C. Parturition
   D. Post-natal development
   E. Suckling
   F. Lactation
3. Offsprings allowed to grow to observe any late effect in:
   A. Behavior
   B. Auditory and visual functions
   C. Reproductive capacity
4. Two or three species—a non-rodent (some require one to be)—for embryotoxicity

mation is to be included in the labeling of all prescription drugs:

Category A: Those drugs that have shown no fetal risk in properly conducted studies in pregnant women; hence, if used when indicated, it is justifiable to assume that any risk to the fetus is small.

Category B: Those drugs in which animal experiments have shown no fetal risk and adequate studies in women are not available; or some risk was observed in animal studies, but not confirmed through controlled studies in human pregnancy.

Category C: Those drugs causing adverse fetal effects in animals, without controlled studies available in women; or where animal and human studies are not available.

Category D: Those drugs which have demonstrated some fetal risk in the human yet because of their benefits are acceptable for use. Patients receiving such drugs should be informed of the risks involved.

Category X: Those drugs shown to be associated with fetal abnormalities by animal or human studies, where the risks clearly outweigh the benefits of the drug. Such drugs are contraindicated in pregnancy.

Information regarding the possible embryotoxicity of drugs in the human comes from several sources: animal studies, epidemiologic surveys, and case studies.

Animal studies represent the underpinning for teratologic evaluation of drugs. Their principal drawback is species specificity. Even within the same species the findings can vary with the particular strain of animals tested. Hence, a particular compound can cause fetal anomalies in animals, but not in man—and the opposite can be true.

Although species specificity is a major stumbling block in extrapolating observations on animals to the human condition, it is by no means the only one. It is probably valid to assume that given the proper circumstances and animal species, most, if not all, drugs will exhibit a degree of teratogenicity. In some, but not all, instances the teratogenic dose of a drug lies between that which produces no apparent effect and that which is lethal to the embryo or fetus. This distinction, however, is not uniformly clear.

Expressed differently, not all doses of a given drug are necessarily teratogenic; hence, teratogenicity is not only a function of the chemical structure but also of the dose. This raises the problem of establishing an acceptable standard for selecting the "appropriate" dose for teratogenic evaluation, and of its relationship to the therapeutic amounts used in the human. Confusing the issue further is the fact that the teratogenic response to a particular compound can vary with the route of administration, and in association with concomitant drugs.

The above remarks notwithstanding, animal testing is an essential and valuable process in the assessment of drug embryotoxicity. Significantly, we are unaware of any epidemic of congenital malformations attributable to maternal drug intake since the thalidomide experience.

Epidemiologic surveys can either be prospective or retrospective. They can describe an observed change over a span of time. In prospective studies a group of exposed (E) and unexposed (UE) subjects are followed to determine the incidence of anomalies in each group and the relative risk, calculated by dividing the incidence of E by that of UE. In retrospective studies, the disease is identified: this group of subjects is then compared with an appropriately selected control group and the incidence of exposure determined for each group. Epidemiologic studies are often difficult to interpret. The sample size may be too small to exclude fortuitous occurrence unless there is a strong and specific teratogenic influence of a particular drug. A large number of subjects are needed before many drugs can be called nonteratogenic as distinct from apparently non-teratogenic. Furthermore, retrospective studies can suffer from biased recall and/or incomplete documentation. Thus, in many instances this approach should be appropriately considered a screening procedure leading to further investigation.

Case reports, while possible sources, usually suffer some major drawbacks, especially if they involve a single or small number of cases. The questions of fortuitousness and biased recall can often be legitimately raised. These apart, other issues remain unanswered, such as incidence among those exposed, the gestational age of sensitivity, the dose-response relationship, and so forth. These and other aspects must be appreciated before clinical policies are formulated based on case reports. Many examples are available of contradictory findings regarding the specific human teratogenicity of a particular drug.

The preceding comments are not meant to detract from the value of these approaches in ferreting out teratogens in man. However, they serve to underline the difficulties encountered in studying teratogens in the human. The value of case reports and epidemiologic studies often lies in drawing attention to a possible framework for documentation. Such reports also provide a basis for assessing relative risks of drug intake to the fetus. It should be remembered that the detection of human environmental teratogens—such as rubella, thalidomide, alcohol—has been largely the result of the alert physician.

Several birth defect surveillance programs have been instituted in the United States (the Center for Disease Control, Congenital Malformations Surveillance, U.S. Department of Health, Education, and Welfare, Public Health Service, January-December 1978). These programs include the Birth Defects Monitoring Program which involves the National Institute of Child Health and Human Development, the Center for Disease Control (CDC), and the Commission on Professional and Hospital Activities; the Metropolitan Atlanta Congenital Defects Program run by the CDC, the Georgia Mental Health Institute, and Emory University School of Medicine; the Birth Defects Prevention Program, Division of Special Health Programs of the Nebraska State Department of Health, and the Surveillance Program of the Health Program Office of the Florida Department of Health and Rehabilitative Services. Among the aims of these programs is monitoring the incidence and types of congenital malformations and providing a registry for epidemiologic and genetic evaluations. Such programs are of great value in detecting warning trends possibly before they reach epidemic proportions, or detecting in the early phases sudden increases in the incidence and types of malformations. Such preliminary work will stimulate a search for possible cause or causes.

References and Recommended Reading

Abdul-Karim, RW (Ed.): Drug therapeutics. Clin Obstet Gynecol 20:361, 1977.

Brown, GW: Berks on fallacy revisited. Am J Dis Child 130:56, 1976.

Doering, PL, Stewart, RB: The extent and character of drug consumption during pregnancy. JAMA 239:843, 1978.

Food and Drug Administration Advisory Committee on Protocols for Safety Evaluations: Panel on Reproduction, Report on Reproduction Studies in the Safety Evaluation of Food Additives and Pesticide Residues. Toxicol Appl Pharmacol 16:264, 1970.

Food and Drug Administration Drug Bulletin: Guidelines for Reproduction Studies for Safety Evaluation of Drugs for Human Use, 1966.

Food and Drug Administration Drug Bulletin, DHEW: Pregnancy Labeling. FDA Drug Bulletin 9:23, 1979.

Forfar, JO, Nelson, MM: Epidemiology of drugs taken by pregnant women: Drugs that may affect the fetus adversely. Clin Pharmacol Therap 14:632, 1973.

Fraser, FC: Prevention of birth defects: How are we doing? Teratology 17:193, 1978.

Greenberg, G, Inman, WHW, Adelstein, AM, Haskey, JC: Maternal drug histories and congenital abnormalities. Br Med J 2:853, 1977.

Heinonen, OP, Slone, D, Shapiro, S: Birth Defects and Drugs in Pregnancy. Littleton, MA, Publishing Sciences Group, 1977, pp. 1-516.

Hill, RM, Craig, JP, Chaney, MD, Tennyson, LM, McCulley, LB: Utilization of over-the-counter drugs during pregnancy. Clin Obstet Gynecol 20:381, 1977.

McBride, WG: The teratogenic action of drugs. Med J. Aust 2:869, 1963.

Nelson, MM, Forfar, JO: Associations between drugs administered during pregnancy and congenital abnormalities of the fetus. Br Med J 1:523, 1971.

Oakley, Jr., GP: Birth defect surveillance in the search for and evaluation of possible human teratogens. In Cytogenetics, Environment, and Malformation Syndromes, U.S. DHEW, 12(5), 1976.

Oakley, Jr., GP: The use of human abortuses in the search for teratogens. In U.S. Department of Health, Education, and Welfare. Methods for Detection of Environmental Agents that Produce Congenital Defects, USDHEW, 1975, p. 189.

Oakley, Jr., GP, Flynt, Jr., W, Falek, A: Community surveillance of birth defects. In USDHEW Genetics Issues in Public Health and Medicine, DHEW, 1978, p. 235.

Peckham, CH, King, RW: A study of intercurrent conditions observed during pregnancy. Am J Obstet Gynecol 87:609, 1963.

Reynolds, JW: The use of drugs in influencing human fetal metabolism. Clin Obstet Gynecol 17(3):95, 1974.

2

GENERAL PRINCIPLES OF DRUG TRANSFER, METABOLISM, AND EFFECTS

TRANSFER

The principal route of drug transfer to the fetus is via the placenta. Prior to its formation, drugs may reach the developing embryo through the *oviductal* and *uterine luminal secretions*. Drugs appear in these secretions most likely as a result of diffusion rather than by way of a specific transport mechanism. The rate of transfer varies with the molecular weight, lipid solubility, and degree of ionization of the drug. At times the concentration of the drug in the luminal fluids may exceed that in the maternal plasma (e.g., nicotine, isoniazid, caffeine, thiopental). In certain instances the drug can be identified, in more than minimal amounts, in the uterine secretions of pregnant animals only.

The pathway(s) by which drugs present in the luminal secretions enter the blastocyst is/are not entirely clear, although most drugs apparently do so by diffusion. The *rate of transfer* is influenced by the pH of the blastocyst (pH 9.0) and that of the uterine fluid (pH 7.6). Hence, acidic substances are more likely to accumulate in the blastula. The distribution of drugs within the blastula may be uneven, with certain areas showing a higher concentration than others. Clearance of the drug from the early embryo can be slow; thus the drug may remain for some time after the initial exposure, raising the possibility of a carry-over effect into the later stages of development.

The *sensitivity* to drug effects differs in the various regions of the blastula. As a rule, extra-embryonic tissues (e.g., trophoblast) are less severely affected than are those of the embryo. All-in-all, the blastula appears to possess a certain degree of resiliency to the possible noxious influence of drugs. An "all or

11

none" long-term effect seems to operate in most instances, i.e., the blastula either dies or overcomes the damage, resulting in an offspring with no obvious malformations. That this resiliency is not absolute is supported by experimental evidence where, for example, prenatal exposure to DDT can cause decreased birthweight and fetal brain weight.

After its formation, the primary route of drug transfer to the fetus is *via the placenta*. Several mechanisms may be operative, the most common being *diffusion*. By this route the rate of transfer is proportional to the surface area and thickness of the membrane. Energy expenditure is not required, and there is no saturation effect or competition between similar molecules.

Less frequently, substances may cross the placenta by *facilitated diffusion* (e.g., glucose). Very few drugs seem to require an *active* transport mechanism while others leak through the membrane pores. Some drugs reach the fetus mainly after having been converted into the placenta from a precursor. For example, the placenta is not readily permeable to ascorbic acid, but can convert dehydroascorbic acid and ascorbic acid which then is readily transferred to the fetus.

FACTORS INFLUENCING TRANSFER

Placental transfer of drugs is affected by several factors. These are summarized in Table 1.

TABLE 1. FACTORS INFLUENCING PLACENTAL DRUG TRANSFER

1. Maternal Placental Circulation
2. The Concentration of the Drug and its Duration in the Maternal Blood
3. The Concentration Gradient Between Fetal and Maternal Blood
4. Properties of the Drug
   A. Lipid Solubility and Degree of Ionization
   B. Molecular Weight
   C. Spacial Configurations
5. Protein Binding
6. Diffusion Capacity of the Placenta
7. Gestational Age
8. Drug Metabolism by Placenta
9. Fetal Circulation

Maternal Placental Circulation—Changes in maternal placental blood flow influence the amount of substances available for transfer over a given period of time. Hence, an increase in blood flow may favor, whereas a decrease in flow reduce, the amount of drug reaching the fetus per unit time. Theoretically, a reduction in maternal placental blood flow at the time of bolus drug administration to the mother would be of some benefit to the fetus. The disadvantages to the fetus of reduced maternal flow are all too obvious to make the willful reduction in placental flow of any clinical value. Hence, this approach is ill-advised. The principle, however, may be applied when drugs are given intravenously in bolus fashion to women in labor. There is merit to the practice of administering such drugs at the beginning of a uterine contraction. Transfer is hindered during the contraction providing more time for the drug to be distributed in the maternal tissues.

Properties of the Drug—These include *molecular weight, special configuration* (certain isomers cross much more readily), *lipid solubility,* and *degree of ionization.*

The placenta may be considered a lipid membrane. Lipid soluble drugs up to a molecular weight of 1000 diffuse across the placenta with relative ease. Water soluble drugs, on the other hand, cross the placenta much less readily. Drugs with molecular weights less than 600 readily traverse the placenta. Above 600 the rate of diffusion decreases. Most therapeutic drugs have a molecular weight ranging between 250-400.

The rate of drug transfer is inversely proportional to the degree of drug ionization. Non-ionized drugs diffuse more readily. Apparently, the majority of drugs traverse the placenta in the non-ionized state. However, exceptions do occur and even fully ionized drugs do reach the fetus, albeit at a slower rate.

Protein Binding—Drugs bound to plasma proteins do not diffuse across the placenta. Consequently, the higher the affinity for binding, the lower the concentration of the free potentially diffusable molecule. Since it is the non-protein bound drug that influences the diffusion rate, measurements of *total* drug concentrations (protein bound and unbound) may not accurately reflect the diffusion gradient. There are differences in binding affinity between maternal and fetal plasma proteins. Maternal plasma proteins have a higher affinity for phenobarbitone and hydantoin among others, and a lower affinity for salicylates.

pH Differences Between Fetal and Maternal Blood—Since the pH in fetal blood is normally below that of the mother, the degree of ionization of acidic drugs is higher in the maternal blood. Consequently, at equilibration the concentration of such drugs tends to be higher in the maternal blood, whereas the reverse occurs with weak bases. The greater the degree of ionization of the drug, the higher the differential, since it is the non-ionized form of the drug that equilibrates across the placenta. These phenomena may explain the higher level of pethidine in newborn versus maternal blood, whereas the level of barbiturates generally remains lower in fetal blood. There are exceptions to these generalizations—as in the case of basic local anesthetics where the fetal levels are usually below those of the mother.

The Fetal Circulation—The degree of partitioning of umbilical vein blood via the ductus venosus influences the amount of blood reaching the liver which may be capable of metabolizing the drug.

Gestational Age—The rate of transplacental transfer can vary with gestational age, being highest in some instances in early pregnancy.

Placental Metabolism—Although the placenta is capable of metabolizing drugs, it is not a very efficient organ in this respect. It may be stated parenthetically that drug metabolism by the placenta is not necessarily always in the interest of the fetus, since the metabolites may be harmful to the fetus.

Apparently, several factors operate in the transfer of drugs. It should be realized that important as these may be, they are significant principally in acute or short-term drug administration. In chronic maternal drug exposure, the factors influencing the rate of transfer become less significant since sufficient time is available for maternal-fetal equilibration. In acute situations (e.g., bolus administration) the ease or rapidity of drug transfer will be measurably influenced by the preceding considerations, although a particular drug may behave in a manner different from that predicted by its characteristics.

PLACENTAL DRUG METABOLISM

Knowledge is still incomplete regarding the extent of drug metabolism by the placenta. Several known pathways are present, as summarized in Table 2.

TABLE 2. METABOLISM OF DRUGS BY PLACENTA

---

1. Oxidation
   A. Not uniformly demonstrable for all drugs
      1. Poorly oxidized—e.g., codeine, hexobarbital, chlorpromazine
      2. Well oxidized—e.g., amphetamine
   B. May be stimulated or inhibited by certain agents or drugs
      1. Stimulation and/or induction—e.g., maternal smoking
      2. Inhibition—e.g., by carbon monoxide, steroids
2. Reduction—active in placenta
          —requires NADPH
          —modified by malnutrition
3. Hydrolysis—e.g., meperidine
4. Conjugation—e.g., acetylation of PABA

The presence of such pathways, however, is not necessarily a barrier to the potentially harmful effect of drugs. On one hand, drugs may reach the fetus in the unaltered state; on the other hand, the metabolites may be as injurious, if not more, to the fetus than the parent compound.

FETAL DRUG METABOLISM

The human fetus possesses the enzymes necessary to metabolize certain drugs. Other pathways available to the fetus to terminate and/or retard drug influence include storage in body fat, binding to tissue and/or plasma proteins, and excretion via the lungs, kidneys, gut and/or placenta.

Like the placenta, fetal drug metabolism does not necessarily confer safety on the fetus, since the resultant metabolites may be as or more damaging than the parent compound. Furthermore, in the absence of other avenues for elimination, water soluble drugs or hydrophilic metabolites can accumulate in the fetus since their passage across the placenta is compromised. With this in mind, it is not surprising that the pathways for hydroxylation and for certain conjugation reactions are not highly active in the fetus.

Fetal drug metabolism may be by oxidation, reduction, hydrolysis, or conjugation and can occur in several fetal organs such as the liver, adrenals, lungs, intestines and brain. Cytochrome P-450 is present in fetal liver, adrenals and placenta. Probably the best known of these pathways is oxidation by the fetal liver, which, because of the anatomy of the fetal circulation, is a primary recipient of drugs transferred via the placenta. Oxidation reactions may be demonstrable in the first trimester wide variability among fetuses. These enzymes may be stimulated by some agents (e.g., prednisone, cigarette smoke) and inhibited by others (e.g., chlorpromazine). Their properties can differ from similar enzymes present in the adult.

DISTRIBUTION OF DRUGS WITHIN THE FETUS

Data on drug distribution within fetal tissues are primarily based on animal studies. The techniques used include analysis of fetal blood and other tissues, autoradiography, and chronic experiments using indwelling catheterization. It is clear that many of these approaches are either difficult or impossible to use in the human. Consequently, most studies in the human rely on umbilical vein-artery blood measurements, or are carried out at the time of therapeutic abortions.

Drugs and/or their metabolites can be widely distributed in fetal tissues, although their extent and concentration are dependent on several factors such as affinity for binding sites, pH gradients and solubility properties of the drug. Therefore, drugs may have a predilection for certain sites in the fetus such as calcifying tissues (e.g., calcium, fluoride), water compartments (e.g., penicillin, bromide, iodide), tissues with a high lipid content, or organs actively involved in metabolizing the drug. The yolk sac appears to be a favored site for concentrating drugs. As a result of these and other factors, a drug may be rather uniformly distributed in the fetal tissue or show more selective concentrations (e.g., chloroquin in the eye). Certain fetal tissues such as the brain seem to possess a similar (as distinct from a selective) affinity for many drugs. At equilibration the concentration of a particular drug in fetal tissues may exceed, equal, or be lower than that in the mother.

EFFECTS ON REPRODUCTION

About 4% of known or suspected causes of human malformations are attributable to environmental chemicals and drugs (Wilson, J.G., 1977). Thus, despite increased awareness of the possible teratogenic effect of drugs, it appears that drugs taken during pregnancy account for only a small proportion of infants with birth defects. However, the *relative* contribution of environmental agents to the overall incidence of congenital malformations seems slightly on the rise. This may be due, at least in part, to the decrease in the birth rate of genetically malformed children because of abortions resulting from improved prenatal diagnosis.

The potential effect of toxic agents on the process of reproduction extends beyond what has been defined traditionally as "congenital malformations." While the emphasis has been on substances taken during pregnancy, it is possible for drugs to exert a preconception influence by affecting the gametes of either parent.

Such an effect may be death of the gamete, a chromosomal defect and/or one that leads to early embryonic death. Although emphasis is usually placed on drugs ingested by the mother, evidence suggests that drugs taken by the father, such as thalidomide and phenytoin, could affect fetal development. These drugs, as well as methadone, are excreted in the semen of both men and rabbits; and conceivably may contribute to the suggested increase in the incidence of malformations among the offspring of fathers taking thalidomide or on anticonvulsant therapy for epilepsy. Similarly, paternal exposure to certain volatile gases, e.g., vinyl chloride, presumably increases the incidence of spontaneous abortions.

Infrequently, even though a long interval may exist between the administration of a drug and a pregnancy, a fetal effect is demonstrable. Offspring of mothers who had received a dye for gallbladder visualization show marked elevation in their PBI even though the dye may have been given as long as two years prior to conception (Shapiro and Man, 1960).

On the other hand, the outcome of drug exposure during pregnancy may become apparent after birth. Examples include withdrawal symptoms in the newborn exposed in utero to addictive drugs; and the apparent link between vaginal adenocarcinoma and prenatal exposure to diethylstilbestrol. More difficult to evaluate are possible biochemical, physiological, or functional impairments such as decrease in longevity, behavioral, and/or mental processes. Nonetheless, the available evidence suggests that such disturbances are possible.

A summary of the possible effects of drugs on reproduction is provided in Table 3.

Overriding preoccupation with the adverse effects of drugs has overshadowed the fact that some drugs are beneficial to the reproductive process. The field of fetal therapy is still in its embryonic stage but sufficient progress has been made to make the concept viable. The treatment of syphilis during pregnancy not only cures the mother, but also her unborn. Other examples exist where drugs are used during pregnancy solely for the purpose of potential benefit to the fetus. These remarks notwithstanding, the risk-benefit ratio should always be carefully evaluated when drugs are administered to the pregnant woman.

18

TABLE 3. POSSIBLE ADVERSE EFFECTS OF DRUGS ON REPRODUCTION

1. Damage to the gametes: leading to relative or absolute infertility—defective zygotes, unrecognized abortions.
2. Increase in the number of recognized abortions: increase in chromosomal and/or structural anomalies.
3. Alterations in the sex ratios at birth.
4. Fetal growth retardation, deaths, congenital anomalies (minor up to those incompatible with life).
5. Disabilities not recognizable at birth that become apparent later in life.
6. Decreased survival and/or a higher likelihood for malignancies.
7. Withdrawal symptoms in the newborn (e.g., addictive drugs).
8. Interference with the fetal endocrine system (e.g., antithyroid drugs).
9. Enzyme inductions (e.g., phenobarbital, glucocorticoids).
10. Changes in neurotransmitter levels (e.g., chlorpromazine).

FACTORS AFFECTING THE INFLUENCE OF DRUGS ON THE FETUS

The factors influencing the effect of drugs on the fetus are summarized in Table 4.

TABLE 4. FACTORS AFFECTING INFLUENCE OF DRUGS ON FETUS

1. Nature—Dosage and duration of drug treatment
2. Gestational age
3. Genetic makeup of fetus and mother
4. Drug-metabolizing capability of mother
5. Metabolism and clearance of drugs from fetal tissues

Not all drugs are equally teratogenic, and the degree of possible maternal harm is not necesarily linked to the degree of potential fetal harm. Furthermore, a teratogenic dose can be somewhere between that which is lethal and that which is harmless. The duration of drug therapy influences outcome not only by an effect on the cumulative amount of the drug and/or metabolites, but also by the exposure of several systems in various stages of development.

A drug may cause one or more malformations; and similar effects may result from dissimilar drugs. In male fetuses diethylstilbestrol is associated with structural and functional genital anomalies, and in females with vaginal adenosis and adenocarcinoma. Furthermore, the manifestations of a drug can differ depending on the period of gestation. In early pregnancy oral anticoagulants may cause nasal and orthopedic anomalies, while in later pregnancy the increased risk to the fetus seems primarily that of hemorrhage and death. A drug that causes abortion—or lethal anomalies leading to abortion—will obviously not be associated with an increased incidence of anomalies at term. It is the nonlethal developmental abnormalities that may appear at term.

Gestational Age—The process of normal development involves several cellular mechanisms that must occur in an orderly pattern. A disturbance in any one or more aspects of this process could lead to developmental anomalies. Hence, the increasing interest and numerous advances in the study of the cellular processes in normal growth.

The initially totipotential cells soon begin to be committed to various specific pathways of development. An integral part of this process is cellular proliferation (cell division), migration, differentiation, and biochemical and physiologic (i.e., functional) maturation. Though extensive overlap exists, these developmental processes generally occur in the above sequence and do not run simultaneously for all organs and tissues. At any particular gestational age, the extent of morphologic and/or functional development will vary among the various organs. To this extent there are "critical periods" of highest susceptibility to teratogens. All in all, the gestational age of highest vulnerability to structural malformations is the principal period of organogenesis usually defined as between 13-56 days. Within this time-span, intervals of increased vulnerability are present for various organs and/or systems, e.g., 15-25 days for the nervous system, 20-40 days for the heart, and longer periods for the genitalia and teeth. (It should be added, parenthetically, that the vulnerability of the central nervous system lasts throughout the period of pregnancy.)

Prior to the period of major organogenesis, most insults appear to have an all-or-none effect. This is not a universal phenomenon as discussed elsewhere.

During the fetal stage, exposure to drugs can interfere with organ growth and/or functional maturation. Decrease in size of various organs may occur, and the decrease may or may not be proportional. Functional disturbances may result, as in the association of chloroquin and quinine with impaired hearing, tetracycline with yellow staining of the teeth and possible inhibition of bone growth, and the antithyroid drugs with fetal goiter.

The possible *long-term effects* of prenatal drugs on human development (without obvious morphogenic effect) is receiving increasing attention, but solid data are scarce. Experimental studies involving sex hormones, morphine, or amphetamine show that offsprings exposed prenatally to these drugs may show abnormalities in the sexual differentiation of the brain, motor behavior, eye opening, body weight gain, the response of the adrenals to stress, and tolerance to the effect of the drug (morphine) in adulthood. In man, in utero exposure to alcohol and diethylstilbestrol may result in impaired reproductive function, and in the case of alcohol, impaired learning capabilities.

Fetal and Maternal Genotypes—The outcome of identical drug exposure during pregnancy can vary between species and among individuals of the same species. Thus in the human, not all of those exposed to thalidomide had affected offsprings. Similarly, in experimental animals the outcome within the species varies greatly among different genetic strains. Some of the factors responsible for the differences in outcome possibly relate to the efficiency by which the drug is metabolized and eliminated by the mother and/or fetus and the nature of the metabolites.

Interest in the outcome of environmental genetic interactions has extended into the frontiers of molecular biology. Mice fetuses possessing the gene or genes that regulate the metabolism of hydrocarbons by the cell are severely affected when exposed to exogenous hydrocarbons, whereas nonresponsive fetuses exhibit only a slight retardation of their growth (Nebert et al., 1972; Shum et al., 1977). It appears that in the responsive group, it is the resultant metabolites of the hydrocarbons that adversely influence the fetus. Hence, the same system designed to protect the adult from hydrocarbons renders the fetus susceptible to malformations.

Another example is found in the production of cleft palate in mice fetuses exposed to exogenous glucocorticoids. The incidence of the anomaly varies with the strain of mice. The facial mesenchymal cells from resistant strains have a lessened ability to bind cortisone than do those from susceptible strains. Variation in the affinity of binding occurs in physiological concentrations of the hormone (Salomon and Pratt, 1976; Goldman et al., 1977).

References and Recommended Reading

Arena, JM: Drug and chemical effects on mother and child. Pediatr Ann 8:10, 1979.

Chamberlain, GVP, Wilkinson, AW: Placental transfer. Pitman Medical Publishing Co., Kent, England, 1979, pp. 1-212.

Gerber, N, Lynn, RK: Excretion of methadone in semen from methadone addicts; Comparison with blood levels. Life Sci 19:787, 1976.

Goldman, AS, Katsumata, M, Yaffe, SJ et al.: Palatal cytosol cortisol-binding protein associated with cleft palate susceptibility and H-2 genotypes. Nature 265:643, 1977.

Joffe, JM: Influence of drug exposure of the father on perinatal outcome. Clin Perinat 6:21, 1979.

Joffe, JM, Peterson, JM, Smith, DJ et al.: Sub-lethal effects on offspring of male rats treated with methadone before mating. Res Commun Chem Pathol Pharmacol 13:611, 1976.

Kretchmer, N: Perspectives in teratologic research. Teratology 17:203, 1978.

Mirkin, BL et al.: Perinatal Pharmacology and Therapeutics. New York, Academic Press, 1976, pp. 1-429.

Nebert, D, Goujon, F, Gielen, J: Aryl hydrocarbon hydroxylase induction by polycyclic hydrocarbons: A simple autosomal dominant trait in the mouse. Nature (New Biol) 236:107, 1972.

Nishimura, H, Tanimura, T: Pharmacology of the conceptus. In Nishimura, H, Tanimura, T. Clinical Aspects of the Teratogenicity of Drugs, New York, American Elsevier, 1976, p. 49.

Salomon, D, Pratt, R: Glucocorticoid receptors in murine embryonic facial mesenchyme cells. Nature 264:174, 1976.

Shapiro, R, Man, EB: Iophenoxic acid and serum-bound iodine values. JAMA 173:1532, 1960.

Shapiro, S, Hartz, SC, Siskind, V et al.: Anticonvulsants and parental epilepsy in the development of birth defects. Lancet 1:272, 1976.

Shum, S, Lambert, G, Nebert, D: The murine Ah locus and dysmorphogenesis. Pediatr Res 11:529, 1977.

Swanson, BN, Leger, RM, Gordon, WP et al.: Excretion of phenytoin into semen of rabbits and man: Comparison with plasma levels. Drug Metab Disposit 6:70, 1978.

Wilson, JG: Embryotoxicity of drugs in man. In Wilson, JG, Fraser, FC (Eds) Handbook of Teratology, Vol I. New York, Plenum Press, 1977, p. 309.

3

DRUGS AND PREGNANCY OUTCOME

CARDIOVASCULAR DRUGS

Cardiac Glycosides

During labor, maternally administered digoxin readily reaches the fetus. Its concentration in fetal blood remains lower than in maternal blood for the first hour after delivery; thereafter the concentrations are similar. Digoxin binds to maternal proteins and is stored in the placenta. During the first trimester 0.1% or less of maternally administered digitoxin can be detected as unchanged, and 0.33% or less of the metabolites can be found in fetal tissues when examined 3-5 hours after the drug has been administered to the mother. A higher percentage (about 0.8 unchanged compound and 3.5 metabolites) can be found at term, reflecting, at least in part, the increase in fetal mass since the concentration of the digitalis in fetal tissues remains unchanged. It is not clear how much of the metabolites are maternal in origin or are the result of drug metabolism by the fetus. It is probable that digitoxin is metabolized in the fetal liver. Based on its body weight compared to the mother's, the fetus has 2-3 times the maternal concentrations of the drug. The highest concentration of the drug is found in the fetal heart and kidney. Digitoxin is also present in the fetal brain, having thus crossed the blood-brain barrier (Okita et al., 1956).

The possible teratogenic effect of digitalis on the human fetus is poorly understood, and the information scanty. In view of its

Acknowledgment: We gratefully acknowledge the help of Dr. David Clark, Assistant Professor of Pediatrics, State University of New York, Upstate Medical Center, in providing the illustrations included in this chapter.

The sections on Antibiotics, Antithyroids, Methadone, and Disulfiram were co-authored by Dr. Thelma J. Yambao.

ready passage across the placenta and (at least after the first hour) the similarity of maternal and fetal blood concentrations, fetal digitalis toxicity is a possible concomitant of maternal intoxication. The therapeutic value of digitalis in suspected fetal heart failure has not been established.

In summary, one may conclude that if digitalis is a teratogen in humans, it is weakly so when used therapeutically. In view of its maternal benefits, we believe digitalis is a justifiable drug for use, when indicated, during pregnancy.

Propranolol

Propranolol, a β-adrenergic blocker, is used in the treatment of several cardiovascular diseases including cardiac arrhythmias, hypertrophic obstructive cardiomyopathy, hypertension, and thyrotoxicosis. It has been used successfully to correct dysfunctional labor associated with fear and anxiety. Propranolol traverses the placenta in its native form, and the level in umbilical blood approximates that of the mother. Its half-life in adults is between 3-5 hours depending on route of administration.

Fetal and Neonatal Effects

There are conflicting reports about the possible effects of propranolol on the fetus. No apparent increase in congenital malformations occurs, although an association with fetal growth retardation has been established. Neonatal respiratory depression, bradycardia, and hypoglycemia are frequently present. Hyperbilirubinemia, hypocalcemia, and polycythemia have also been described infrequently.

The conflicting reports about possible effects of propranolol on the fetus may be due, at least in part, to the different amounts of the drug taken by the mother and to the time interval between the last dose and delivery. Other factors not standardized for are the influence of the maternal disease itself and of concomitantly administered drugs. Not uncommonly, dosages lower than 160 mg/day have little observable effect on the fetus or newborn. These babies rarely exhibit neonatal respiratory depression or hypoglycemia and their apgar scores are usually high, although small placentas have been described. A strong association seems to exist between higher propranolol dosage and neonatal depression, hypoglycemia, and low apgar ratings. However, this dose-effect relationship is not observed consistently, and neonatal hypoglycemia and depression are to be watched for in infants born to all mothers undergoing propranolol therapy.

The relationship between intrauterine growth retardation (IUGR) and propranolol is less clear. Since many of the diseases for which propranolol is indicated are themselves conducive to IUGR, it is difficult to separate the effect of the disease from that of the drug. Furthermore, this possible association is often cited in case reports which lack appropriate controls for definitive evaluation. Among the mechanisms purported to predispose to IUGR is one mediated via propranolol's β-blockade property. In essence such an effect could lead to an increase in resting myometrial tonus which in turn produces a decrease in intervillous blood flow. Whether this does occur remains to be seen. Nonetheless, IUGR is not a consistent finding with maternal propranolol intake; and although the available evidence does not exclude it, fetal growth retardation appears to occur infrequently.

Infants of propranolol-treated mothers should be considered at risk and managed as such. The bradycardia and hypoglycemia may persist for more than two hours after birth. Propranolol is bound to tissues and is mainly metabolized by the liver. Prolonged maternal exposure to the drug could result in significant amounts being present in fetal tissues. This, coupled with the relative immaturity (compared to adults) of newborn liver (particularly in the premature), could lead to slow elimination of the drug. The effect of propranolol on hepatic blood flow (a fall) could reduce its rate of metabolism further. The lower albumin concentration in the newborn, especially those who are preterm, may lead to a relatively higher concentration of the unbound, and hence potentially more active, drug.

Effect of Indices of Fetal Heart Rate Monitoring

It should be noted that with propranolol, fetuses may not exhibit the classical signs associated with fetal hypoxia. These fetuses may become hypotensive rather than the reverse, and may fail to show a tachycardia once the hypoxic insult is removed. Experimentally, it has been shown that an increase in fetal cardiac output may not occur and fetal death from hypoxia could be accelerated. These findings might be explained by a blockade of the β-receptors in the fetal heart.

Furthermore, under propranolol, other fetal heart changes used as indices for fetal welfare may be altered. The basal fetal heart rate can be lowered and the fetal tachycardia often seen with uterine contractions abolished.

These effects on the fetus may be of clinical relevance primarily in situations which are in themselves conducive to fetal hypoxia. In the absence of impaired intervillous flow the fetus may not demonstrate any ill effects in its growth potential, whereas if intervillous flow is already compromised, the added effect of propranolol could be sufficient to impair fetal growth.

In summary, when maternal considerations dictate the need for treatment with propranolol, we believe that its use during pregnancy is justified. The prospective mother and father should be fully apprised of the potential risks involved.

Disopyramide

Disopyramide is an antiarrhythmic drug whose action is similar to that of quinidine. It is particularly useful in the treatment of ventricular arrhythmias. Recently Shaxted and Milton (1979) reported on a patient with ventricular tachycardia treated with disopyramide 200 mg every 8 hours from the 26th week of pregnancy. The pregnancy progressed normally and the fetal heart rate showed no abnormalities. At delivery, disopyramide levels in maternal and cord blood were 2.3 and 0.9 mg/l, respectively. The newborn was of normal weight and exhibited no anomalies. Significantly, intrapartal fetal bradycardia occurred during an episode of hypertonic uterine contractions. This indicated that the fetal heart rate responded appropriately in the presence of the drug in fetal blood (albeit at levels probably below the adult therapeutic range). Much wider experience is undoubtedly needed with this drug during pregnancy.

References and Recommended Reading

Anderson, PO, Salter, FJ: Propranolol therapy during pregnancy and lactation. Am J Cardiol 37:325, 1976. (Letter to the Editor)

Bharadwaja, K, Promisloff, R: Clinical pharmacology of propranolol. Drug Ther (Hosp) March:22, 1977.

Bott-Kanner, G, Schweitzer, A, Reisner, SH, Joel-Cohen, SJ, Rosenfeld, JB: Propranolol and hydralazine in the management of essential hypertension in pregnancy. Br J Obstet Gynaecol 87:110, 1980.

Cottrill, CM, McAllister, Jr., RG, Gettes, L, Noonan, JA: Propranolol therapy during pregnancy, labor, and delivery: Evidence for transplacental drug transfer and impaired neonatal drug disposition. J Pediatr 91:812, 1977.

Elliahou, HE, Silverberg, DS, Reisin, E, Romem, I, Mashiach, S, Serr, DM: Propranolol for the treatment of hypertension in pregnancy. Br J Obstet Gynaecol 85:431, 1978.

Fiddler, GI: Propranolol and pregnancy. Lancet 2:722, 1974. (Letter to the Editor)

Gilani, SH, Silvestri, A: The effect of propranolol upon chick embryo cardiogenesis. Expl Cell Biol 45:158, 1977.

Gladstone, GR, Hordof, A, Gersony, WM: Propranolol administration during pregnancy: Effects on the fetus. J Pediatr 86:962, 1975.

Habib, A, McCarthy, JS: Effects on the neonate of propranolol administered during pregnancy. J Pediatr 91:808, 1977.

Kolibash, AJ, Ruiz, DE, Lewis, RP: Idiopathic hypertrophic subaortic stenosis in pregnancy. Ann Intern Med 82:791, 1975.

Levitan, AA, Manion, JC: Propranolol therapy during pregnancy and lactation. Am J Cardiol 32:247, 1973. (Letter to the Editor)

Lieberman, BA, Stirrat, GM, Cohen, SL, Beard, RW, Pinker, GD, Belsey, E: The possible adverse effect of propranolol on the fetus in pregnancies complicated by severe hypertension. Br J Obstet Gynaecol 85:678, 1978.

Mitrani, A, Oettinger, M, Abinader, EG, Sharf, M, Klein, A: Use of propranolol in dysfunctional labour. Br J Obstet Gynaecol 82:651, 1975.

Ohnhaus, EE, Spring, P, Dettli, L: Protein binding of digoxin in human serum. Europ J Clin Pharmacol 5:34, 1972.

Okita, GT, Plotz, EJ, Davis, ME: Placental transfer of radioactive digitoxin in pregnant women and its fetal distribution. Circ Res 4:376, 1956.

Padeletti, L, Porciani, MC, Scimone, G: Placental transfer of digoxin (beta-methyl-digoxin) in man. Int J Clin Pharmacol & Biopharm 17:82, 1979.

Pruyn, SC, Phelan, JP, Buchanan, GC: Long-term propranolol therapy in pregnancy: Maternal and fetal outcome. Am J Obstet Gynecol 135:485, 1979.

Reed, RL, Cheney, CB, Fearon, RE, Hook, R, Hehre, FW: Propranolol therapy throughout pregnancy: A case report. Anesth Analgesia 53:214, 1974.

Rogers, MC, Willerson, JT, Goldblatt, A, Smith, TW: Serum digoxin concentrations in the human fetus, neonate and infant. N Engl J Med 287:1010, 1972.

Rosen, TS, Lin, M, Spector, S, Rosen, MR: Maternal, fetal and neonatal effects of chronic propranolol administration in the rat. J Pharmacol Exp Ther 208:118, 1979.

Sabom, MB, Curry, Jr., RC, Wise, DE: Propranolol therapy during pregnancy in a patient with idiopathic hypertrophic subaortic stenosis: Is it safe? So Med J 71:328, 1978.

Shoenfeld, N, Epstein, O, Nemesh, L, Rosen, M, Atsmon, A: Effects of propranolol during pregnancy and development of rats. I. Adverse effects during pregnancy. Pediatr Res 12:747, 1978.

Shand, DG: Propranolol: Resolving problems in usage. Drug Therap (Hosp) Aug:52, 1978.

Shaxted, EJ, Milton, PJ: Disopyramide in pregnancy: A case report. Curr Med Res Opin 6:70, 1979.

Sherman, JL, Jr., Locke, RV: Transplacental neonatal digitalis intoxication. Am J Cardiol 6:834, 1960.

Silber, DL, Durnin, RE: Intrauterine atrial tachycardia. Am J Dis Child 117:722, 1969.

Tcherdakoff, PH, Colliard, M, Berrard, E, Kreft, C: Propranolol in hypertension during pregnancy. Br Med J 2:670, 1978.

Van Petten, GR: Pharmacology and the fetus. Br Med Bull 31:75, 1975.

ANTIHYPERTENSIVES

Chronic maternal hypertension increases the incidence of fetal and maternal complications during pregnancy. The magnitude of this increase is directly related to the severity of the hypertension. Medicinal treatment of the hypertension is beneficial to the mother, but controversy exists as to an improvement in fetal welfare. In addition, as with other drugs, the prospect of potential fetal effects from the medication enters into consideration.

Methyldopa

In 1968 Leather and co-workers reported on the outcome of drug therapy in 100 patients with moderate (diastolic pressure of 90-99 mm Hg) or severe (diastolic pressure of 100 mm Hg or greater) hypertension. Fifty-two women were treated with methyldopa (0.5-2 g/day), bendrofluazide 5-10 mg/day, potassium supplements, and when needed, other hypotensive drugs such as hydralazine. The remaining patients served as controls. The results suggested that when the hypertension was present prior to 20 weeks of gestation, an increase in both the duration of pregnancy and birth weight occurred accompanied by a decrease in perinatal morbidity and mortality. No adverse fetal effects ascribed to treatment were recorded in this group.

In 1964, Hans and Kopelman utilized methyldopa, along with hydrochlorothiazide or bendrofluazide and phenobarbitone, to treat 15 preeclamptic patients at 28-37 weeks of gestation. The dose of methyldopa varied between 250-500 mg 3-4 times daily depending on the blood pressure response. Therapy averaged 19 days (range 7-47 days). No untoward effects were found in the surviving babies. Subsequently, Kincaid-Smith et al. (1966) reported on 32 severely hypertensive patients treated with methyldopa during their pregnancy. The majority were treated for 3-6 months; 5 patients received the medication during the first trimester. Seven patients also received reserpine or chlorothiazide. Several patients had associated renal or other disease. The authors describe the beneficial effect of methyldopa in controlling maternal hypertension. Although they state that there were no "significant abnormalities" in the infants, four of the neonates had umbilical hernias and one a slight clitoral enlargement. The specific maternal regimen of therapy for these five newborn is not recorded, although the authors later state that there was no evidence of ill effects to the fetus of mothers treated during the first trimester.

The benefits and safety of methyldopa were examined in a controlled prospective study involving 242 pregnant women

(Redman et al., 1976). Methyldopa and, where necessary, other drugs were employed. Although no specific effect of treatment on birth weight, length of gestation, or newborn maturity was observed, an overall improvement in outcome occurred, partly due to a lower rate of mid-trimester abortions. The cause of the decrease in the abortion rate is unclear. No adverse fetal effects were reported. The authors conclude that pending further work, the use of methyldopa during pregnancy should be based on maternal indications, and that the drug was safe for both mother and fetus. Birth weights, when corrected for gestational age, were similar in treated and untreated hypertensives, although the mean head circumference was slightly higher in the latter (34.6 cm ± 1.34 vs. 34.16 cm ± 1.68) (Mutch et al., 1977). It appears that this difference cannot be accounted for by a tendency toward lower birth weight in the treated patient.

Head circumference did not correlate with either the amount or duration of methyldopa treatment, but appeared to relate to the time at which patients entered and hence began therapy (16-20 weeks). Infants of mothers beginning treatment before this period were not affected even though the medication was continued throughout. However, the authors introduced a word of caution in the interpretation of their results. Follow-up of children up to one year of life showed that at one year of age there were no differences in either weight or head circumference (Mutch et al., 1977). More infants in the untreated hypertensive group showed abnormal or questionable gross motor abilities, and neurologic status.

A follow-up assessment showed that the average head circumference of boys (but not girls) at four years of age was slightly reduced, but the possibility that this was a chance occurrence was raised (Ounstead et al., 1980). In any case, there was no correlation between head circumference and the total developmental score. Children of treated mothers had consistently higher mean scores in the developmental sectors examined than did those of untreated mothers. The authors conclude that hypertension in pregnancy is associated with a slight delay in developmental aspects of the children and that therapy with methyldopa may reduce this effect.

Methyldopa crosses the placenta and reaches levels in total plasma similar to those in the mother. The concentration in amniotic fluid may be higher.

The available evidence suggests that the use of methyldopa in pregnancy is safe for both mother and fetus, and may even be of some benefit to the offspring of hypertensive pregnant women. Patients on methyldopa are to be followed for possible side effects, and we should note that a positive Coombs test may be recorded. However, in the studies reviewed, there are only a few patients who are less than 10 weeks' pregnant. So we cannot conclude that the available evidence negates a teratogenic effect of methyldopa when administered during the embryonic period. This aspect awaits specific documentation. Furthermore, the possible causal relationship of methyldopa with reduced fetal head circumference cannot be totally dismissed at present even though it appears that catch-up growth does occur postnatally. The explanation for this possible association is not known, and indeed the authors insert a word of caution when discussing the possible cause. Any explanation must take into account the singular observation of the relationship of decrease in head circumference to period of gestation when patients first entered the study. It is not easy to explain why a relationship was not observed if the medications were taken earlier and continued through the specified period. Clearly, many more studies are needed. We look forward to continuing longitudinal studies on children exposed to methyldopa in utero.

Hydralazine

Hydralazine, a peripheral vasodilator, is a phthalazine derivative. Until the rise in use of methyldopa it was probably the most commonly used agent of its class in the management of chronic and acute hypertensive diseases in pregnant women. The controversy concerning fetal benefits of lowering the maternal blood pressure is not entirely resolved, although there is general agreement that properly controlled reduction in blood pressure is beneficial to the mother and possibly the fetus as well. Hydralazine increases cardiac output and produces tachycardia. The concomitant use of propranolol may allow a decrease in the effective individual dose of both drugs, and reduce the sympathomimetic side effects of hydralazine.

The blood pressure response to intravenously administered hydralazine occurs within 15 minutes. Side effects occur rather frequently and include nausea, vomiting, diarrhea, anorexia, palpitation, and headaches. Another drawback is occasional inefficacy.

In view of its effect on cardiac output, hydralazine would not appear to be the drug of choice in pregnant women with left ventricular outflow obstruction such as idiopathic hypertrophic subaortic stenosis. Although such patients can go through pregnancy safely, the disease can be hazardous and propranolol is better suited for symptomatic patients. Its prophylactic use in labor and delivery seems warranted.

There is no evidence to implicate hydralazine in the formation of congenital malformations in the human. However, the drug has been used primarily after the first 10 weeks of pregnancy. We are unaware of controlled human studies addressing themselves to the safety of hydralazine when given during the embryonic stage of development.

Reserpine

Reserpine (Rauwolfia serpentina) is a hypotensive agent that produces its effect by acting predominantly on the central nervous system. Contrary to other hypotensive agents, reserpine slows the heart rate.

Reserpine crosses the placenta. Newborn of reserpine-exposed mothers can exhibit several side effects, most commonly nasal congestion and lethargy. Other effects include excessive secretions, bradycardia, hypothermia, and decreased responsiveness of the Moro reflex.

The nasal congestion, which may last up to 6 days, is a major problem for the newborn since they are predominantly nose breathers. This coupled with the lethargy can lead to problems in ventilation, hence infants of reserpine-treated mothers must be observed closely and meticulously. The lethargy is usually gone in less than 24 hours.

Not all the newborn of reserpine-treated mothers show side effects, and it is not clear what determines the presence or absence of such side effects. There is no clear-cut dose-effect relationship, nor an absolute correlation with maternal side effects. In multiple gestation one twin may be affected and the other not. The nasal congestion effect of reserpine seems less marked in prematures.

The predominant experience with reserpine during pregnancy is in the management of the acute toxemias. Consequently, the data apply to short-term exposure principally in the 3rd trimester.

There is a dearth of information on pregnancy outcome in long-term and first trimester exposure to reserpine, and therefore its degree of teratogenicity, if any, in the human remains unanswered; it is our impression at this time that reserpine is not a strong teratogen in the human.

Diuretics

The role of diuretics in the therapy of pregnant women has had a checkered career. Their value has been broadly challenged, particularly in the management of the acute toxemias of pregnancy; and indeed many investigators suspect that they could be of harm. Nevertheless, diuretics are occasionally indicated during pregnancy, and thus fetal considerations come into play.

Despite their widespread use, there is a dearth of well controlled studies to evaluate the effect of diuretics on the fetus. Many diuretic drugs are clearly teratogenic in animals, and the carbonic anhydrase inhibitors, with few exceptions, produce a fairly specific form of congenital anomaly in rodents. The timing of drug exposure during the pregnancy is important. Congenital anomalies have been produced experimentally with other diuretic agents.

The available evidence in the human does not implicate the use of diuretics during pregnancy with congenital malformations. In one retrospective study the incidence of congenital malformations among women who had taken chlorothiazide during pregnancy was not increased (McBride, 1963). However, the number of women exposed to diuretics during the first trimester was not specified. In controlled trials using chlorothiazide and methylchlorothiazide during pregnancy, the drugs were given after the first trimester and for relatively short periods of time. The primary focus of the studies was the effect of such agents on preeclampsia, hypertension, or edema. The question of teratogenicity was not addressed (Menzies, 1964; Mackay and Khoo, 1969).

Chlorothiazide rapidly crosses the placenta and its levels in fetal and maternal blood are comparable. This raises the possibility that the drug may have a diuretic effect on the fetus. The drug is not detectable in fetal blood if the maternal dose was administered eight or more hours prior to delivery.

There is an intimate relationship between the osmotic pressure and electrolyte composition of maternal and fetal blood. Factors that alter maternal blood osmotic pressure result in similar changes in fetal blood. Consequently, any maternal electrolyte imbalance incidental to diuretics may be reflected in electrolyte changes in fetal blood. Persistent fetal bradycardia has been described as associated with maternal hypokalemia (Anderson and Hanson, 1974). The fetal heart rate returned to normal following KCl infusion to the mother. This plus the low level of potassium in the amniotic fluid are presumptive evidence that the fetal bradycardia was due to fetal hypokalemia.

In rats, prenatal salt deprivation is associated with lower birth size and a high hematocrit and hyponatremia in the pups (Mouw

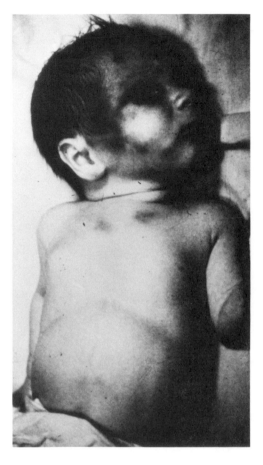

Fig. 1. Neonatal thrombocyto-penia—Areas of ecchymosis on the chest and face. Mother had received thiazide diuretics dur-ing the pregnancy.

et al., 1978). Significantly, there is an increase in the water intake of these animals when fully grown. This is not due to changes in plasma electrolytes or osmolarity, and hence may represent an effect on the fetal brain. We are not aware of comparable studies in the human, although the possibility of fetal growth retarda-tion as a sequela of chronic diuretic therapy has been raised (Lindberg, 1979). One may speculate that contraction of the blood volume leading to reduction in intervillous perfusion is one of the mechanisms involved.

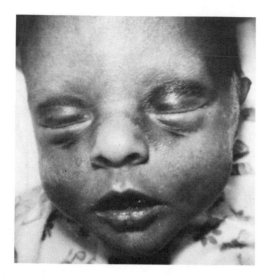

Fig. 2. Another example of neonatal thrombocytopenia associated with maternal intake of thiazide diuretics.

Neonatal hemolysis and thrombocytopenia causing various degrees of hemorrhage have been associated with prenatal thiazide intake. Though not conclusive, the available evidence points to a possible relationship between methyclothiazide, bendroflumethiazide, hydrochlorothiazide, and chlorothiazide taken during pregnancy, and hematologic alterations in the neonate. In many instances other drugs have been taken concomitantly, which complicates the issue of a cause-effect relationship. The thrombocytopenia in the newborn appears to be due to decreased megakaryocyte production; and other evidence of bone marrow depression may occur such as reticulocytopenia, leukopenia, or pancytopenia. The mechanism of this bone marrow depression is unclear, but it apparently is not immunologic in nature, and the mothers need not show any concomitant hematologic abnormalities. Not all infants of thiazide-treated mothers demonstrate hematologic abnormalities (their prevalence is essentially undetermined), nor is the relationship to dosage and duration of drug therapy clear.

In summary, there is no evidence to incriminate diuretics as teratogens in the human. However, the preponderance of diuretic use during pregnancy occurs after the first trimester and therefore the data do not in effect exclude an adverse effect of the drugs during embryogenesis. Thiazides may on occasion result in bone marrow depression in the newborn, and this possibility should be kept in mind at delivery in women exposed to the drug.

In view of the trend to discourage the chronic use of diuretics during pregnancy, the physician nowadays should encounter the problem infrequently. In the event that they are used, attention to maternal, and by implication fetal, electrolyte balance is essential. It would seem prudent when possible to discontinue the diuretics two or more weeks prior to an anticipated delivery.

Diazoxide

Diazoxide, a benzothiadiazine without diuretic activity, exerts its vasodilator effect by acting directly on the smooth muscles. It should not be given to patients sensitive to thiazides. It effectively lowers the blood pressure in preeclampsia, and appears safe for both mother and fetus. Given intravenously, it produces a rapid hypotensive response. Both cardiac output and pulse rate increase. It seems to produce a proportionate fall in both the systolic and diastolic blood pressures. The maximum hypotensive response is reached within 5-15 minutes and in most instances lasts up to 4 hours; the dose may be repeated. Maternal and newborn hyperglycemia frequently occurs, but this appears to be of no consequence to mother or fetus. Myometrial relaxation and decrease in the frequency of uterine contractions may occur; the latter can be augmented with oxytocin.

Although the effect of lowering the blood pressure with diazoxide therapy on the intervillous circulation in the human is unknown, the fetal heart rate in most instances remains normal. This may be taken as indirect evidence that should there be a decrease in intervillous flow, it is not of the magnitude to produce recognizable fetal hypoxia. Indeed, with the vasodilation and increased cardiac output, an increase in intervillous perfusion seems likely. However, the standard dose (300 mg bolus IV) may produce severe maternal hypotension, and the fetal heart may become tachycardic with type II decelerations. Therefore, the fetal heart rate response may relate to the severity of the hypotension. These responses, as may be expected, are more readily apparent in growth-retarded fetuses. It should be noted that rarely has diazoxide been used as the sole agent in preeclamptic patients, so the observed effects may to some extent reflect synergistic responses.

It should be noted that preeclamptics have contracted blood volume—a fact to be kept in mind when hypotensive agents are used. Since diazoxide is rapidly bound to plasma proteins, the drug, unlike hydralazine, cannot be titrated slowly to produce the desired effect. The pros and cons of this property are still argued. Diazoxide can displace coumarin derivatives from serum albumin, and hence the anticoagulant dose may have to be readjusted. Diazoxide crosses the placenta and can be identified in infant blood 24 hours after delivery. In animals, diazoxide can destroy the islet cells of the fetus (Boulos et al., 1971).

Oxprenolol

Oxprenolol is a β-adrenergic receptor blocker. Gallery et al. (1978) used the drug in 19 pregnant women with moderately severe hypertension. The mean gestational age at beginning therapy was 29 weeks, and the maximal daily dose used was 480 mg. In approximately one-third of the patients, hydralazine was added to achieve the desired blood pressure response (i.e., a sitting diastolic of 80 mmHg or less). Delivery occurred at 38 ± 0.4 weeks. No fetal or newborn complications were attributable to oxprenolol. Specifically, there were no intrapartal fetal heart changes attributable to the drug, and none of the infants exhibited bradycardia, hypoglycemia or respiratory depression. The Apgar scores were normal. Therapy appeared to increase birth weight compared with untreated hypertensives, although it was still below the projected birth weight of a normal population. The authors conclude that lowering the blood pressure had no detrimental fetal effects. On the contrary, it appeared to be beneficial; this suggests that more rigorous attention be given to lowering the diastolic blood pressure.

In a subsequent paper these authors compared oxprenolol with methyldopa for the treatment of hypertension during pregnancy (Gallery et al., 1979). As in their previous work, each drug dosage was adjusted to maintain a sitting diastolic blood pressure of 80 mmHg or less, and hydralazine was added to each drug when indicated. Initiation of therapy, excluding 10 women who had been receiving treatment before conception, averaged 21 ± 1.8 (S.E.) and 32 ± 0.8 (S.E.) weeks, respectively, for the two drugs. Mean age of delivery for the oxprenolol-treated group was 38 ± 0.4 (S.E.) weeks vs. 37.5 ± 0.6 for the methyldopa group.

A comparable level of blood pressure control was achieved in both groups. However, the mean birth weight in the oxprenolol group was similar to controls, and significantly greater (average

400 g) than in the methyldopa group. Apgar scores were similar in both groups and there were no intrauterine deaths. However, blood sugar levels of infants in the former group were normal but significantly higher than in the methyldopa-exposed babies, two of whom became hypoglycemic and required treatment.

There was a significant correlation between blood pressure (diastolic) control and plasma volume in the oxprenolol group, a correlation less well defined in the methyldopa group. The lower the diastolic pressure the higher the plasma volume. Plasma volume directly correlated with birth weight in the oxprenolol group. It was concluded that oxprenolol was associated with a greater expansion of the blood volume, which in turn improved intervillous circulation and led to enhancement of fetal growth. The effect on plasma volume was less pronounced (statistically not significant) with methyldopa.

Obviously the issue of teratogenesis was not addressed in these studies. However, the results are encouraging and if confirmed, could indicate that oxprenolol is a safe and effective agent for use in hypertensive states during pregnancy after the first trimester. Its fetal safety in earlier use remains to be determined.

Metoprolol

Metoprolol is another adrenergic β-receptor blocker that has been tried in the management of hypertensive disease in pregnancy. While β-adrenergic receptor blockers share a common hypotensive effect, their other effects are not necessarily comparable. Metoprolol is a selective β_1 blocker and as such may have some advantages when used during pregnancy.

Sandström (1978) treated 101 pregnant women with essential or pregnancy-induced hypertension. Metoprolol was given in dosages not exceeding 400 mg per day. Another group of patients received hydralazine. Hydralazine was also given to some patients in the metoprolol group. The average time of delivery was around 38 weeks.

The mean reduction in maternal blood pressure was higher in the metoprolol-treated mothers. The average birth weight was similar in both groups, although there appeared to be a higher tendency for small-for-date babies in the hydralazine group. However, there were fewer intrauterine and neonatal deaths among the metoprolol group.

Although metoprolol crossed the placenta, its concentration in fetal plasma was lower than that in the mother. The majority of babies had a heart rate above 100 beats per minute, although the mother showed a reduction in pulse rate as a result of metoprolol treatment. The authors find merit in the combination of metoprolol and hydralazine for the management of hypertension during pregnancy.

As with other drugs in the same category, the teratogenic potential of metoprolol when administered during the first trimester has not been ascertained.

Labetalol

Labetalol is an α and β-adrenoreceptor antagonist. Its use in hypertensive diseases (essential or pregnancy-induced) during pregnancy was reported by Michael (1979) and Lamming and Symonds (1979). Labetalol was used for 1-12 weeks, but it is not clear if any of the patients were between 4-10 weeks' pregnant when therapy was initiated. The drug given orally proved effective in lowering blood pressure in both chronic and pregnancy-induced hypertension and was without apparent harmful maternal or fetal effects. A careful examination of the newborn retinae was performed. Labetalol crosses the placenta, but its concentration in cord blood is below that in maternal blood. No fetal heart changes ascribable to the drug were detected.

A possible beneficial effect of labetalol on fetal pulmonary maturation has been noted (Michael, 1979). In this series no patient had to be delivered prior to fetal lung maturation. A comparison of this finding with that following the use of other hypotensive agents suggested that the effect on fetal pulmonary maturation was not shared by all antihypertensive drugs. The clinical findings are consistent with the data in rabbits, demonstrating fetal pulmonary surfactant enhancement following prenatal labetalol exposure (Nicholas et al., 1978).

The teratogenic potential of labetalol in the human has not been evaluated.

Clonidine

Clonidine, an imidazoline derivative, is an effective agent for the treatment of hypertension. When given intravenously, it has a rapid hypotensive effect that reaches its maximum within 20-30 minutes and lasts from 1-2 hours.

Its side effects include drowsiness, dry mouth and pallor. Clonidine is effective in lowering the blood pressure in acute hypertension during pregnancy, and its employment for that purpose during labor has produced no observable adverse effects on the newborn. Rebound hypertension can occur after clonidine withdrawal. This and the unavailability of studies on its chronic use in pregnancy which demonstrate an advantage over other available agents makes its use during pregnancy inadvisable at this time.

OTHER ANTIHYPERTENSIVE AGENTS

Bethanidine

Bethanidine, an adrenergic neuron blocking agent, may be used to manage acute toxemias of pregnancy. It has a rapid action; patients must be hospitalized for therapy. The initial dose of bethanidine, 10 mg 4 times per day orally, may be increased to achieve the desired response in blood pressure. Bethanidine, along with guanethidine (which acts by preventing norepinephrine release from nerve endings), has low lipid solubility, but this should not be taken to indicate that these drugs do not cross the placenta. Both drugs reduce maternal cardiac output, renal blood flow, as well as the blood flow to other organs. Diarrhea and postural hypotension may occur. We believe these drugs should only be used selectively during pregnancy.

Ganglionic Blocking Agents

These are contraindicated during pregnancy. They offer no known advantages over other available agents. They cross the placenta and cause meconium ileus in the newborn.

Veratrum Alkaloides

Historically, these drugs were among the first available hypotensive agents. Currently, there are no indications for their use in pregnancy.

References and Recommended Reading

Altstatt, LB: Transplacental hyponatremia in the newborn infant. J Pediatr 66:985, 1965.

Anderson, GG, Hanson, TM: Chronic fetal bradycardia: Possible association with hypokalemia. Obstet Gynecol 44:896, 1974.

Arias, F, Zamora, J: Antihypertensive treatment and pregnancy outcome in patients with mild chronic hypertension. Obstet Gynecol 53:489, 1979.

Asslai, NS: Thiazide diuretics in toxemia of pregnancy. JAMA 174:887, 1960. (Editorial)

Battaglia, F, Prystowsky, H, Smisson, C, Hellegers, A, Bruns, P: Fetal blood studies. XII. The effect of the administration of fluids intravenously to mothers upon the concentrations of water and electrolytes in plasma of human fetuses. Pediatrics 25:2, 1960.

Berkowitz, RL: Anti-hypertensive drugs in the pregnant patient. Obstet Gynecol Surv 35:191, 1980.

Boulos, BM, Davis, LE, Almond, CH, et al.: Placental transfer of diazoxide and its hazardous effect on the newborn. J Clin Pharmacol 11:206, 1971.

Budnick, IS, Leikin, S, Hoeck, LE: Effect in the newborn infant of reserpine administered ante partum. Am J Dis Child 90:286, 1955.

Chamberlain, GVP, Lewis, PJ, DeSwiet, M, Bulpitt, CJ: How obstetricians manage hypertension in pregnancy. Br Med J 1:626, 1978.

Davies, AM: Epidemiology of the hypertensive disorders of pregnancy. Bull WHO 57:373, 1979.

Desmond, MM, Rogers, SF, Lindley, JE, Moyer, JH: Management of toxemia of pregnancy with reserpine. II. The newborn infant. Obstet Gynecol 10:140, 1957.

Editorial: Unclassified mental retardation. Lancet 1:250, 1979.

Gallery, EDM, Saunders, DM, Hunyor, SN, Gyory, AZ: Hypertension in pregnancy. Med J Aust 1:540, 1978.

Gallery, EDM, Saunders, DM, Hunyor, SN, Gyory, AZ: Improvement in foetal growth with treatment of maternal hypertension in pregnancy. Clin Sci Mole Med 55:359S, 1978.

Gallery, EDM, Saunders, DM, Hunyor, SN, Gyory, AZ: Randomised comparison of methyldopa and oxprenolol for treatment of hypertension in pregnancy. Br Med J 1:1591, 1979.

Garnet, JD: Placental transfer of chlorothiazide. Obstet Gynecol 21:123, 1963.

Hans, SF, Kopelman, H: Methyldopa in treatment of severe toxaemia of pregnancy. Br Med J 1:736, 1964.

Harley, JD, Robin, H, Robertson, SEJ: Thiazide-induced neonatal haemolysis. Br Med J 1:696, 1964.

Johansson, S, Andersson, RGG, Wikberg, J: Mechanical and metabolic effects of diazoxide in rat uterus. Acta Pharmacol Toxicol 41:328, 1977.

Johnston, CI, Aickin, DR: The control of high blood pressure during labour with clonidine ("Catapres"). Med J Aust 2:132, 1971.

Kaplan, NM: Antihypertensive drugs in combination. Effects of methyldopa on thiazide-induced changes in renal hemodynamics and plasma renin activity. Arch Intern Med 135:660, 1975.

Keith, TA III: Hypertension crisis. Recognition and management. JAMA 237:1570, 1977.

Kincaid-Smith, P, Bullen, M, Mills, J: Prolonged use of methyldopa in severe hypertension in pregnancy. Br Med J 1:274, 1966.

Lamming, GD, Symonds, EM: Use of labetalol and methyldopa in pregnancy-induced hypertension. Br J Clin Pharmacol 8:217S, 1979.

Leather, HM, Humphreys, DM, Baker, P, Chadd, MA: A controlled trial of hypotensive agents in hypertension in pregnancy. Lancet 2:488, 1968.

Lindberg, BS: Salt, diuretics and pregnancy. Gynecol Obstet Invest 10:145, 1979.

Lindheimer, MD, Katz, AI: Sodium and diuretics in pregnancy. N Eng J Med 288:891, 1973.

Lundborg, P: Fetal effects of antihypertensive drugs. Acta Medica Scand 628(Suppl):95, 1979.

Mackay, EV, Khoo, SK: Clinical and laboratory study of a new diuretic agent ("Vectren") in pregnancy: A comparison with a diuretic agent in current use ("Enduron"). Med J Aust 1:607, 1969.

Martin, JD: A critical survey of drugs used in the treatment of hypertensive crises of pregnancy. Med J Aust 2:252, 1974.

McBride, WG: The teratogenic action of drugs. Med J Aust 2:689, 1963.

Menzies, DN: Controlled trial of chlorothiazide in treatment of early pre-eclampsia. Br Med J 1:739, 1964.

Merenstein, GB, O'Loughlin, EP, Plunket, DC: Effects of maternal thiazides on platelet counts of newborn infants. J Pediatr 76:766, 1970.

Michael, CA: Treatment of hypertension arising in pregnancy. Drugs 15:317, 1978.

Michael, CA: Use of labetalol in the treatment of severe hypertension during pregnancy. Br J Clin Pharmacol 8:211S, 1979.

Milner, RDG, Choukjey, S: Effects of fetal exposure to diazoxide in man. Arch Dis Child 47:537, 1972.

Moar, VA, Jefferies, MA, Mutch, LMM, Ounsted, MK, Redman, CWG: Neonatal head circumference and the treatment of maternal hypertension. Br J Obstet Gynaecol 85:933, 1978.

Morris, JA, Arce, JJ, Hamilton, CJ, Davidson, EC, Maidman, JE, Clark, JH, Bloom, RS: The management of severe preeclampsia with intravenous diazoxide. Obstet Gynecol 49:675, 1977.

Mouw, DR, Vander, AJ, Wagner, J: Effects of prenatal and early postnatal sodium deprivation on subsequent adult thirst and salt preference in rats. Am J Physiol 234:F59, 1978.

Mutch, LMM, Moar, VA, Ounsted, MK, Redman, CWG: Hypertension during pregnancy, with and without specific hypotensive treatment. Early Hum Dev 1:59, 1977.

Neuman, J, Weiss, B, Rabello, Y, Cabal, L, Freeman, RK: Diazoxide for the acute control of severe hypertension complicating pregnancy: A pilot study. Obstet Gynecol 53:50S, 1979.

Nicholas, TE, Lugg, MA, Johnson, RG: Maternal administration of salbutamol and labetalol increases the amount of alveolar surfactant in lung of the day 27 fetal rabbit. Proc Aust Physiol Pharmacol Soc 9:146P, 1978.

Nuwayhid, B, Brinkman, CR, Katchen, B, Symchowicz, S, Martinek, BS, Asslai, NS: Maternal and fetal hemodynamic effects of diazoxide. Obstet Gynecol 46:197, 1975.

Ounsted, MK, Moar, VA, Good, FJ, Redman, CWG: Hypertension during pregnancy with and without specific treatment; the development of the children at the age of four years. Br J Obstet Gynaecol 87:19, 1980.

Perkins, RP: Treatment of toxemia of pregnancy. JAMA 238:2143, 1977. (Letter)

Pritchard, JA, Walley, PJ: Severe hypokalemia due to prolonged adminis-tration ot chlorothiazide during pregnancy. Am J Obstet Gynecol 81:1241, 1961.

Redman, CWG, Beilin, LJ, Bonnar, J, Ounsted, MK: Fetal outcome in trial of antihypertensive treatment in pregnancy. Lancet 2:753, 1976.

Ring, G, Krames, E, Shnider, SM, Wallis, KL, Levinson, G: Comparison of nitroprusside and hydralazine in hypertensive pregnant ewes. Obstet Gynecol 50:598, 1977.

Roberts, JM, Perloff, DL: Hypertension and the obstetrician-gynecologist. Am J Obstet Gynecol 127:316, 1977.

Rodriguez, SU, Leikin, SL, Hiller, MC: Neonatal thrombocytopenia associated with antepartum administration of thiazide drugs. N Eng J Med 270:881, 1964.

Sandström, B: Antihypertensive treatment with the adrenergic beta-recep-tor blocker metoprolol during pregnancy. Gynecol Obstet Invest 9:195, 1978.

Sobel, DE: Fetal damage due to ECT, insulin coma, chlorpromazine, or re-serpine. Arch Gen Psych 2:606, 1960.

Vink, GJ, Moodley, J, Philpott, RH: Effect of dihydralazine on the fetus in the treatment of maternal hypertension. Obstet Gynecol 55:519, 1980.

ANTICOAGULANTS

The need for anticoagulants during pregnancy is not in-frequent. The principal indications are venous thromboembolic disease and cardiac valve prosthesis.

Because of the increased coagulability of the blood during pregnancy, and the occasional necessity for prolonged periods of inactivity, it is not surprising that the incidence and severity of venous thromboembolic disease during pregnancy would be increased over that of suitably matched controls. Venous throm-boembolism is still a cause of maternal death, although the risk is materially reduced by anticoagulant therapy.

Patients with prosthetic heart valve replacements are predis-posed to systemic embolization. This propensity for emboli for-mation may be expected to increase during pregnancy. Changes in valve designs have diminished but not removed the risk; con-sequently, these patients are placed under continuous anti-coagulant therapy to minimize the risk of embolization.

The most commonly used anticoagulant drugs during pregnancy are heparin and anti-vitamin K agents. The role of antiplatelet agents, especially in pregnancy, has not yet been defined. Throm-bolytic agents are contraindicated during pregnancy, except pos-sibly as a life-saving measure in massive thromboembolism.

Heparin

Because of its large molecular weight and negative charge, heparin, as far as can be determined, does not cross the placenta, nor to our knowledge has it been implicated in any fetal teratogenesis. From these standpoints heparin may be considered the safest anticoagulant available for use during pregnancy. It is the drug of choice during the first 12 weeks of pregnancy. Its major drawback is that parenteral administration is necessary, although in long-term therapy most patients can easily be taught the technique of subcutaneous self-administration.

Warfarin

Warfarin is the coumarin agent most frequently used in the management of thromboembolic diseases. It is of low molecular weight, and traverses the placenta with ease. Because of the immaturity of its liver enzymes, the fetus probably is less capable of metabolizing the drug.

Exposure to warfarin during pregnancy is suspected of causing a number of congenital anomalies. Exposure during the first trimester is thought to be associated with fetal growth retardation, nasal cartilage hypoplasia, frontal bossing, stippling of the bones, and brachydactyl. Stippling occurs most frequently in the vertebral column, followed by the long bones and ankles. Other less frequently described features include mental retardation, cataracts, and optic atrophy. Such effects may be dose-related to the amount of warfarin taken by the mother. Some of the features described resemble those of the Conradi-Hunermann syndrome.

Although warfarin has mainly been implicated in congenital malformations when given during the first trimester of pregnancy, there is suggestive though less well-documented evidence that warfarin given after the first trimester may also be teratogenic, causing micro- or hydro-cephaly, cerebral agenesis, and optic atrophy. The mechanism(s) by which warfarin induces congenital anomalies is unknown. Speculation centers around the occurrence of microhemorrhages at the affected site leading to disturbances in development. It may be difficult to reconcile all of the findings with such a mechanism.

Despite these observations, warfarin cannot be designated as definitely teratogenic in man on current evidence. The evidence available is based on reports which utilize small sample sizes, and in many instances, the patients were receiving other medications. Congenital anomalies are not apparent in every instance where warfarin is used during the first trimester of pregnancy. Nevertheless, it seems prudent at this time to consider warfarin as possibly teratogenic.

There are other adverse effects of warfarin administered during pregnancy, including a higher incidence of abortions and stillbirths. An increased risk of fetal hemorrhage has been suggested, although this may be present only if the medication is carried to term and/or excessive dosages are employed. The fetuses seem particularly vulnerable to bleeding during labor.

RECOMMENDATIONS

We therefore make the following recommendations:

1. Pregnant patients must not be denied anticoagulant therapy if needed.

2. Anti-vitamin K compounds should not be used during the first trimester, or for 3-4 weeks prior to term. During these times heparin is the drug of choice.

3. The problem becomes much more complex when chronic anticoagulation during the second and early third trimesters is considered. Two approaches based on current information seem reasonable: properly monitored oral (warfarin) therapy, or self-administered subcutaneous heparin. Of the two approaches we favor and recommend the latter—expense and patient inconvenience notwithstanding. In the event that the patient cannot tolerate heparin or learn the technique of self-administration, carefully monitored warfarin therapy is to be employed. In any case, as with all other medications, a frank and comprehensive discussion of the risks involved should be held with the patient.

4. In the event that labor occurs while the patient is taking warfarin, it should be discontinued and vitamin K (5 mg) given intravenously, with fresh frozen plasma. This is another drawback to warfarin since the onset of labor is not always predictable. The length of time needed for the disappearance of fetal effects of coumadin is unknown, but it could be as long as 14 days. Vitamin K should be administered to the newborn.

References and Recommended Reading

Barr, Jr., M, Burdi, AR: Warfarin-associated embryopathy in a 17-week old abortus. Teratology 14:129, 1976.

Berg, D, Meltzer, V: Outpatient management of placental insufficiency with heparin. J Perinat Med 6:141, 1978.

Editorial. Anticoagulants and heart valve replacement in pregnancy. Br Med J 1:1047, 1977.

Gericke, GS, van der Walt, A, de Jong, G: Another phenocopy for chondrodysplasia punctata in addition to warfarin embryopathy? S Afr Med J 54:6, 1978.

Hall, JG, Pauli, RM, Wilson, KM: Maternal and fetal sequelae of anticoagulation during pregnancy. Am J Med 68:122, 1980.

Hirsh, J, Cade, JF, Gallus, AS: Anticoagulants in pregnancy: A review of indications and complications. Am Heart J 83:301, 1972.

Kakkar, VV, Bentley, PG: Letter: Long-term self-administered subcutaneous heparin in pregnancy. Br Med J 2:124, 1978.

Larsen, JF, Jacobsen, B, Holm, HH, Pedersen, JF, Mantoni, M: Intrauterine injection of vitamin K before the delivery during anticoagulant therapy of the mother. Acta Obstet Gynecol Scand 57:227, 1978.

Raivio, O, Ikonen, E, Saarikoski, S: Fetal risks due to warfarin therapy during pregnancy. Acta Paediatr Scand 66:735, 1977.

Robinson, MJ, Pash, J, Grimwade, J, Campbell, J: Letter: Fetal warfarin syndrome. Med J of Aust 1:157, 1978.

Shaul, WL, Hall, JG: Multiple congenital anomalies associated with oral anticoagulants. Am J Obstet Gynecol 127:191, 1977.

Spearing, G, Fraser, I, Turner, G, Dixon, G: Long-term self-administered subcutaneous heparin in pregnancy. Br Med J 1:1457, 1978.

Warkany, J: Warfarin embryopathy. Teratology 14:205, 1976.

ANTICONVULSANTS

Epilepsy and Pregnancy

The incidence of obstetrical complications, such as hyperemesis, vaginal bleeding, and the number of intervention procedures needed, appears to be increased in epileptic women, as are prematurity, intrauterine growth retardation, and perinatal morbidity and mortality. In addition, it is generally agreed that the incidence of congenital malformations is higher in the offspring of epileptic women. What is at issue is whether this increase is due to the disease itself, the drugs employed in its treatment, or to both. The controversy is still not settled. (Most of the studies on this point have been retrospectives of reports on relatively few patients.)

The effect of pregnancy on seizure frequency varies. A small percentage of epileptic women experience a decrease in seizure frequency. The cause of this lowered frequency is not clear, but may relate in part to better patient compliance with medication intake. Roughly one-half of the remaining patients experience an increase in seizure frequency, while it remains unaltered in the other half. As a rule, the greater the seizure frequency prior to conception, the more likely the frequency will increase during pregnancy. Recognizing the possibility of increased seizure frequency is important not only because of maternal hazards but because it may jeopardize fetal welfare. Seizures can be associated with increased fetal and neonatal morbidity and mortality, especially during and following status epilepticus. Such episodes are accompanied by a significant degree of maternal hypoxia and acidosis.

In view of the heightened potential for harm to the mother and her fetus from epileptic seizures, it is clear that antiepileptic medications should be maintained during pregnancy in those patients prone to seizure attacks. The question of possible drug teratogenicity then assumes practical significance. By comparing the prevalence of congenital anomalies among treated and untreated epileptics, and the prevalence of congenital anomalies in the general population, the answer should emerge.

No uniform opinion exists as to the incidence of congenital anomalies in nontreated epileptic patients, although the balance of evidence seems to favor an increase. Genetic predisposition is a possibility since the prevalence of congenital anomalies appears greater in the relatives of epileptics, as in the offspring of epileptic fathers. Furthermore, by virtue of the resultant hypoxia and acidosis, seizures—particularly those occurring during early pregnancy—may be conducive to malformations. These considerations are important when evaluating the possible teratogenic effect of anticonvulsants.

The malformations commonly associated with epilepsy include cleft lip and palate and congenital heart disease. The incidence of the former appears to be increased by five-fold or greater; the latter by two to three-fold. Other anomalies have been described, but the correlation with epilepsy is less clear.

Anticonvulsants and Congenital Malformations

An association between antiepileptic drugs and "specific" fetal anomalies has been proposed, but we are not aware of any large well-controlled prospective studies that address themselves to definitely proving or disproving this issue. The strongest association appears to be with trimethadione, but hydantoin and phenobarbital have also been implicated. The congenital defects presumably associated with each medication are in many respects similar to each other and to those associated with maternal alcoholism. The anomalies reportedly related to hydantoin include physical and mental retardation, craniofacial malformations (variations in head size, shape, widening of the fontanelles, epicanthal folds, short nose, wide nasal bridge, strabismus, prominent ears) and limb deformities. Anomalies associated with trimethadione and phenobarbital include physical and mental developmental disturbances, features similar to those described above, and cardiac and occular anomalies. To our knowledge, carbamazepine has not been implicated so far as a teratogen. Congenital glaucoma, optic nerve hypoplasia, and neonatal hypocalcemia may relate to epilepsy and/or its treatment. The rate of anomalies appears to be highest in treated vs. nontreated epileptics and to correlate with dosage, number of drugs used, and number of seizures. Besides these developmental anomalies, newborn of mothers treated with phenytoin, barbiturates, or trimethadione may exhibit hemorrhagic tendencies, most commonly in the cranium, thorax, or abdomen, due to deficiencies in vitamin K clotting factors. These are preventable by administering vitamin K to the newborn. Barbiturate withdrawal symptoms which can remain for an extensive period after birth may occur in the newborn.

To date there is no evidence that children or women treated with antiepileptic drugs are more prone to develop malignancies. The possibility that phenytoin administration during pregnancy is associated with an increased likelihood of developing malignancies in the offspring was raised by the report of Blattner et al. (1977) of a malignant mesenchymoma in a patient with cleft lip and palate. The authors also referred to two children with neuroblastomas of mothers who had received phenobarbitone and phenytoin during pregnancy. Despite the lack of firm evidence, children exposed in utero to these agents should be followed closely for evidence of malignancy.

Clearance During Pregnancy

Antiepileptic drugs readily cross the placenta. The concentrations of phenytoin, carbamazepine, and phenobarbital in fetal blood are similar to those in maternal blood. The maternal plasma levels of phenytoin and phenobarbital decrease during pregnancy probably as a result of increased clearance. Folic acid, given to pregnant women, may also contribute to the lowering of plasma phenytoin levels. These and other aspects, e.g., the volume of fetal and placental tissues, malabsorption, and the increase in the vascular and extravascular spaces can result in a higher antiepileptic drug requirement during pregnancy. Phenytoin plasma protein binding is not altered significantly.

As stated previously, plasma clearance of phenytoin during pregnancy is increased and returns to nonpregnant values within several weeks after delivery. No significant change in plasma clearance of phenobarbital occurs. The increased plasma clearance of phenytoin seems to correlate with a higher rate of seizure frequency, hence, monitoring maternal plasma phenytoin levels is indicated during pregnancy to help maintain the appropriate dose. The increased clearance cannot be accounted for by changes in protein binding; in part it may reflect the increased volume (maternal, fetal, and placental, fluid compartments and tissues) available for drug distribution and possibly, increased drug metabolism during pregnancy. It is unlikely that increased renal excretion is a factor, since presumably it is the unbound drug that is excreted, and there is no change in plasma protein binding properties during pregnancy. Indeed, measurement of urinary phenytoin may serve as an index of the adequacy of the therapeutic regimen, since low or absent urinary phenytoin appears to correlate with increased seizure frequency during pregnancy.

It is possible that the metabolism of phenytoin during pregnancy is influenced by the marked rise in steroids that occurs. Estrogens can reduce the half-life of phenytoin. However, it is also possible that—due to the competition of steroids and phenytoin for existing metabolic pathways—the plasma level of the drug may increase (albeit temporarily) during early pregnancy. The significance of this possibility lies in the suggestion that high levels of phenytoin may correlate with the development of congenital malformations.

RECOMMENDATIONS

The following recommendations seem appropriate at this time. Epileptic women should be advised of the possible increased risk of malformations, and that this effect may be due to the disease, the drug used in treatment, or to both. Despite such risk, there will not be any demonstrable defects in the children of most epileptics. If feasible, it is prudent to discontinue anticonvulsant medication prior to conception and to counsel epileptic women accordingly. Patients requiring antiepileptic medication should be apprised of the facts involved and share in the decision-making process. Discontinuation of indicated medication is not a justifiable alternative. Patients who have been seizure-free without medication may become pregnant without resumption of the antiepileptic drugs unless needed. At present, we recommend that trimethadione not be employed during pregnancy, and an alternative drug used. The experience with carbamazepine in pregnancy is still not extensive, and although the evidence so far has not implicated it in fetal malformation, wider experience is needed before its safety can be assessed. At this time we believe there is less compelling evidence for the teratogenicity of phenobarbital than with hydantoin; when possible, it is recommended that the former be substituted for the latter during pregnancy. Combinations of antiepileptic drugs are best avoided during pregnancy. It is advisable to monitor the drug levels in the maternal blood, particularly during the first ten weeks of pregnancy.

Women taking medication who seek advice late in pregnancy should be informed of the known risks and continued on the medication, since presumably most of the potential harm would already have occurred. Whether maternal supplementation with folic acid in an attempt to reduce the possible teratogenic risk is warranted is still a matter for conjecture.

References and Recommended Reading

AAP Committee on Drugs: Anticonvulsants and pregnancy. January 1979. Prepared by the AAP Committee on Obstetrics: Maternal and Fetal Medicine.

AM Acad of Pediatrics Committee on Drugs: Anticonvulsants and pregnancy. Pediatrics 63:331, 1979.

Annegers, JF, Elveback, R, Hauser, W, Kurland, T: Do anticonvulsants have a teratogenic effect? Arch Neurol 31:364, 1974.

Blattner, WA, Henson, DE, Young, RC, Fraumeni, Jr., JF: Malignant mesenchymoma and birth defects. JAMA 238:334, 1977.

Bleyer, WA, Skinner, AL: Fatal neonatal hemorrhage after maternal anticonvulsant therapy. JAMA 235:626, 1976.

Bodendorfer, TW: Fetal effects of anticonvulsant drugs and seizure disorders. Drug Intell Clin Pharm 12:14, 1978.

Boreus, LO, Jalling, B, Wallin, A: Plasma concentrations of phenobarbital in mother and child after combined prenatal and postnatal administration for prophylaxis of hyperbilirubinemia. J Pediatr 93:695, 1978.

Bustamante, SA: Fetal hydantoin syndrome in triplets. Am J Dis Child 132:978, 1978.

50

Desmond, MM, Schwanecke, RP, Wilson, GS, Yasunaga, S, Burgdorff, I: Maternal barbiturate utilization and neonatal withdrawal symptomatology. J Pediatr 80:190, 1972.

Fabro, S, Brown, NA: Teratogenic potential of anticonvulsants. N Eng J Med 300:1280, 1979. (Letter)

Fedrick, J: Epilepsy and pregnancy: A report from the Oxford Record Linkage Study. Br Med J 2:442, 1973.

Fernandez-Pol, JA, Zaninovich, AA: Effects of administration of estrogen or diphenylhydantoin on the kinetics of diphenylhydantoin in man. J Nucl Med 16:305, 1975.

Friis, B, Sardemann, H: Neonatal hypocalcaemia after intrauterine exposure to anticonvulsant drugs. Arch Dis Child 52:239, 1977.

German, J, Ehlers, KH, Kowal, A, DeGeorge, FV, Engle, MA, Passarge, E: Possible teratogenicity of trimethadione and paramethadione. Lancet 2:261, 1970.

Hanson, JW, Smith, DW: The fetal hydantoin syndrome. J Pediatr 87:285, 1975.

Hill, RM: Fetal malformations and antiepileptic drugs. Am J Dis Child 130:923, 1976.

Hill, RM, Verniaud, WM, Horning, MG, McCulley, LB, Morgan, NF: Infants exposed in utero to antiepileptic drugs. Am J Dis Child 127:645, 1974.

Hill, RM, Verniaud, WM, Morgan, F, Nowlin, J, Glazener, LJ, Horning, MG: Urinary excretion of phenobarbital in a neonate having withdrawal symptoms. Am J Dis Child 131:546, 1977.

Hoyt, CS, Billson, FA: Maternal anticonvulsants and optic nerve hypoplasia. Br J Ophthal 62:3, 1978.

Janz, D: The teratogenic risk of antiepileptic drugs. Epilepsia 16:159, 1975.

Lander, CM, Edwards, VE, Eadie, MJ, Tyrer, JH: Plasma anticonvulsant concentrations during pregnancy. Neurology 27:128, 1977.

Landon, MJ, Kirkley, M: Metabolism of diphenylhydantoin (phenytoin) during pregnancy. Br J Obstet Gynaecol 86:125, 1979.

Loughnan, PM, Gold, H, Vance, JC: Phenytoin teratogenicity in man. Lancet 1:70, 1973.

Loughnan, PM, Greenwald, A, Purton, WW, Aranda, JV, Watters, G, Neims, AH: Pharmacokinetic observations of phenytoin disposition in the newborn and young infant. Arch Dis Child 52:302, 1977.

McElhatton, PR, Sullivan, FM, Toseland, PA: Teratogenic activity and metabolism of primidone in the mouse. Epilepsia 18:1, 1977.

Meadow, R: The teratogenicity of epilepsy. Dev Med Child Neurol 16:375, 1974.

Meadow, SR: Glaucoma, maternal epilepsy, and anticonvulsant drugs. J Pediatr 90:499, 1977. (Letter)

Meyer, JG: The teratological effects of anticonvulsants and the effects on pregnancy and birth. Europ Neurol 10:179, 1973.

Monson, RR, Rosenberg, L, Hartz, SC, Shapiro, S, Heinonen, OP, Slone, D: Diphenylhydantoin and selected congenital malformations. N Eng J Med 289:1049, 1973.

Montouris, GD, Fenichel, GM, McLain, Jr., LW: The pregnant epileptic. Arch Neurol 36:601, 1979.

Mygind, KI, Dam, M, Christiansen, J: Phenytoin and phenobarbitone plasma clearance during pregnancy. Acta Neurol Scand 54:160, 1976.

Nakane, Y: Congenital malformation among infants of epileptic mothers treated during pregnancy. The report of a collaborative study group in Japan. Folia Psychiatr Neurol Japonica 33:363, 1979.

Orringer, CE, Eustace, JC, Wunsch, CD, Gardner, LB: Natural history of lactic acidosis after grand-mal seizures. N Eng J Med 297:796, 1977.

Ramsay, R, Strauss, RG, Wilder, BJ, Willmore, LJ: Status epilepticus in pregnancy: Effect of phenytoin malabsorption on seizure control. Neurology 28:85, 1978.

Richens, A, Houghton, GW: Use of sulthiame during pregnancy. Br Med J 2:544, 1973.

Sanders, BM, Draper, GJ: Childhood cancer and drugs in pregnancy. Br Med J 1:718, 1979.

Segal, S, Anyan, WR, Cohen, SN, Freeman, J, Hill, RM, Kauffman, RE, Pruitt, AW, Shinefield, HR, Vickers, SM: Anticonvulsants and pregnancy. Pediatr 63:331, 1979.

Seino, M, Miyakoshi, M: Teratogenic risks of antiepileptic drugs in respect to the type of epilepsy. Folia Psychiat Neurol 33:379, 1979.

Smith, DW: Teratogenicity of anticonvulsive medications. Am J Dis Child 131:1337, 1977.

Stumpf, DA, Frost, M: Seizures, anticonvulsants, and pregnancy. Am J Dis Child 132:746, 1978.

Tanimura, T: Evaluation of the teratogenicity of anticonvulsants. Folia Psychiat Neurol 33:371, 1979.

Waziri, M, Ionasescu, V, Zellweger, H: Teratogenic effect of anticonvulsant drugs. Am J Dis Child 130:1022, 1976.

Zackai, EH, Mellman, WJ, Neiderer, B, Hanson, JW: The fetal trimethadione syndrome. J Pediatr 87:280, 1975.

ANTIBIOTICS

Penicillin

Despite its wide use, penicillin has not been implicated as a teratogenic drug in humans.

Penicillin and the synthetic analogues (methicillin, dicloxacillin, ampicillin) are readily transferred to the fetus and amniotic fluid throughout gestation. Penicillin reaches the fetus in sufficient amounts to be of therapeutic value in the management of congenital syphilis.

Blecher and co-workers (1966) administered ampicillin (500 mg orally every six hours for five days) to pregnant women at term. Peak maternal blood levels were reached 2-3 hours after each dose. Amniotic fluid levels taken 3-5 hours after the third dose varied from 0.42 µg/ml to 5.1 µg/ml and were on the average four times higher than the corresponding maternal serum levels. The concentration of ampicillin in the cord blood ranged from 0.24 to 2.0 µg/ml. The relationship to maternal serum levels at delivery varied—in 61% of the cases, the cord levels were less.

Bray (1966) infused 500 mg of ampicillin over a 10-15 minute period to normal gravidas in early labor. Serial amniotic fluid and maternal blood samples were obtained at varying intervals as were maternal and cord blood samples at delivery. Peak maternal concentrations (26.5 µg/ml) occurred immediately following the infusion, falling to levels of 1.0 µg/ml within two hours and becoming undetectable at five hours. The levels of ampicillin in the maternal blood one hour after infusion were similar to the peak levels in the cord blood. Concentrations of ampicillin in cord blood reached maximum levels averaging 6.6 µg/ml in one hour, thereafter falling gradually to undetectable values after 12 hours. Amniotic fluid levels continued to rise as maternal serum levels declined and reached a maximum concentration of 5.20 µg/ml in 8 hours. This indicates that the antibiotic is slowly released into the amniotic fluid compartment possibly via the fetal kidneys. This suggestion is compatible with the observation that lower amniotic fluid concentrations are reached when similar amounts of ampicillin are infused in pregnancies with intrauterine fetal death; furthermore, with equivalent maternal doses, the levels of ampicillin reached in amniotic fluid during the first trimester are below those found in the amniotic fluid of women at term.

Similar distribution patterns to those noted with ampicillin are found for other synthetic penicillins. The percentages of dicloxacillin, methicillin, and ampicillin bound to maternal serum proteins are 97%, 40% and 26%, respectively. Since the degree of protein binding affects the diffusion gradient across the placenta, the rate of transfer is lowest for dicloxacillin and highest for ampicillin.

From the available evidence, it appears that with respect to embryotoxicity, penicillin and ampicillin are among the safest antibiotics to use during pregnancy. At present, insufficient information is available regarding the teratogenicity of other synthetic penicillins.

Erythromycin
Erythromycin is a suitable alternative for patients allergic to penicillin. To date, no fetal harm has been ascribed to the use of erythromycin during pregnancy.

A great deal of variability in maternal serum levels of erythromycin occurs following oral usage, probably secondary to an altered gastrointestinal motility which may delay absorption and increase the exposure to destruction by gastric acid. Although hepatic dysfunction has been associated with other erythromycin preparations, hepatotoxicity appears most frequently with erythromycin estolate. The hepatotoxicity of the latter has been described in both pregnant and nonpregnant patients. McCormack et al. (1977) reported that approximately 10-15% of pregnant women receiving erythromycin estolate for 3 or more weeks developed subclinical hepatic toxicity. This is reversible following cessation of treatment. In view of the above, it is probably advisable not to use erythromycin estolate during pregnancy.

Erythromycin does cross the placental barrier although its rate of transfer has not been studied. In general, the concentrations of fetal blood are below those of maternal blood. Philipson et al. (1973) determined fetal tissue levels of erythromycin after single and multiple oral doses of the estolate form were given to pregnant women undergoing abortions. The concentration of the drug in fetal tissue levels approximately 2-8 hours after a single dose equivalent to 500 mg of erythromycin base was: .02 μg/ml in fetal blood; .01 μg/ml in the amniotic fluid and 0.41 μg/ml in the fetal liver. The peak maternal blood concentration averaged 2.55 μg/ml. After multiple doses, the average concentrations in maternal and fetal blood were 4.94 μg/ml and .06 μg/ml, respectively. Erythromycin was also demonstrable in the fetal liver, spleen, lung, brain, muscle and bone. The highest concentration was in the fetal liver which suggests that the organ can concentrate erythromycin.

The lack of uniformity of erythromycin absorption from the gastrointestinal tract raises important considerations in the therapy of a pregnant woman. Multiple oral doses are necessary in order to achieve effective maternal plasma levels. Although erythromycin crosses the placenta and can be demonstrated in the amniotic fluid, the levels achieved in the fetal tissue may be insufficient to treat fetal infections. Congenital syphilis can be present despite adequate maternal therapy with oral erythromycin. Consequently, it is recommended that newborns of syphilitic mothers who were treated with oral erythromycin should be considered partially treated, and further diagnostic and therapeutic measures instituted. The value of intravenous erythromycin alone or in combination in the management of syphilis during pregnancy warrants investigation.

Cephalosporins

A large number of oral and parenteral cephalosporins are presently available with comparable antimicrobial activity. The cephalosporins include cephalothin, cephaloridine, cephapirin, cephacetrile, cefazolin, cefamandole, cefoxitin, cephalexin, cephaloglycin, cefadroxil, and cefaclor.

In adults, *cefazolin* reaches a higher blood level, has a longer half-life and a higher affinity for protein-binding than most cephalosporins. Similarly, it is excreted by the kidneys at a lower rate with a lesser degree of renal toxicity (Bernard et al., 1977).

The distribution of *cefazolin* in maternal and umbilical cord sera and fetal tissues was studied in pregnant women undergoing abortions during the first and second trimesters. After intravenous administration (14 mg/kg) of cefazolin, peak maternal levels were observed within two hours. The drug was detected in cord serum from 45 minutes up to 10 hours after injection, with values ranging from 1-11 μg/ml. The drug reached higher concentrations in fetuses greater than 14 weeks' gestation. Fetal urine examined 2-19½ hours afterward showed the drug to be present in concentrations ranging from 0.4-4.9 μg/ml. The drug was detectable only in the amniotic fluid from second trimester pregnancies but was not found in fetal brain, cerebrospinal fluid, lung, liver or kidney (Bernard and associates, 1977).

Cephalothin rapidly crosses the placenta. Soon after an intravenous dose of 1000 mg, maternal and fetal sera levels in one study reached 30.2 and 12.5 μg/ml, respectively (MacAulay and Charles, 1968). After five hours, the level in maternal serum was 0.08 μg/ml, and 0.67 μg/ml in cord serum. The drug was detectable in the amniotic fluid 15 minutes after injection at levels of 0.25 μg/ml.

From the available data and our limited experience, it would seem that cephalosporins may be used at least during the last trimester of pregnancy, and are well-tolerated by the pregnant patient. As in other newer antibiotics, the question of teratogenicity cannot be answered at this time.

Aminoglycosides

The aminoglycosides possess ototoxic and nephrotoxic properties in adults. Streptomycin causes predominantly vestibular disturbances while dihydrostreptomycin, kanamycin and neomycin mainly produce hearing damage.

Streptomycin and *dihydrostreptomycin* are utilized in the treatment of active tuberculosis. Both are transferred across the placenta. The concentration of these compounds in fetal blood appears to vary with the interval of time between maternal administration and sampling of cord blood.

Conway and Birt (1965) examined 17 children (aged 6-13 years) whose mothers had received streptomycin or dihydrostreptomycin at some time during pregnancy. Minor abnormalities of the eighth nerve function were found in 8 children. Six had abnormal caloric tests without complete loss of labyrinthine function and only two of these had abnormal audiograms (i.e., labyrinthine damage without deafness). Rasmussen (1969) examined 36 children 2-15 years of age and found slight unilateral sensory neural high tone hearing loss in only one child. All had normal vestibular functions. In both of these studies, many of the patients had received other drugs like isoniazid and para-aminosalicylate. Furthermore, these studies were retrospective and did not include appropriate control samples to elucidate the incidence of defects noted in unexposed children.

Varpela et al. (1969) also found a low incidence of nondisabling inner ear defects among children (5 years or older) born to mothers who had received either streptomycin or dihydrostreptomycin at various stages of pregnancy including the period of organogenesis. One cochlear defect was noted among forty children. Vestibular studies done on 34 of these children disclosed two with some defects. Although Varpela and co-workers did not compare their findings with appropriately matched controls, they do indicate that the observed defects are found in children who have not been exposed to streptomycin preparations.

Although the above study does not prove that the observed inner ear defects in the children were due to their in utero exposure to streptomycin or dihydrostreptomycin, the findings do not exclude a cause-effect relationship. Nonetheless, it appears that the resulting effects are largely nondisabling, and that there is no obvious relationship either to the stage of pregnancy when the drug was used or to the total amount given to the mother. However, these issues are not completely resolved and it would be prudent to avoid excessive dosages, particularly in patients where elimination of the drug is compromised (e.g., abnormal renal function). Furthermore, it may be that the children with streptomycin-induced inner ear defects may be vulnerable to further injury from additional use of drugs with ototoxic properties.

Other than the potential effects on the eighth nerve, we are unaware of data linking the streptomycins to congenital human malformations.

The other aminoglycosides—kanamycin, gentamicin, neo-mycin, tobramycin, and amikacin have similar potential ototox-ic properties. All have been shown to traverse the placenta.

After a single dose (40 mg IM) of *gentamicin* given to pregnant women prior to delivery, peak maternal levels of 3.65 μg/ml were attained within 30 mintues. These levels decreased rapidly and after 3-6 hours, the mean maternal level of 0.78 μg/ml was the same as that in the cord. Mean levels in cord blood were 1.25 μg/ml at 1-2 hours which corresponded to 34.2% of the maternal blood value (Yoshioka et al., 1972). Similar results have been obtained by Kauffman et al. (1975) who studied placental transfer during the midtrimester (18-23 weeks) in patients undergoing abortion. Gentamicin was given intravenously (80 mg) followed by an infusion of 18.5 mg/hr 2-6 hours prior to surgery. The average maternal serum concentrations ranged from 2.1-6.2 μg/ml. Fetal central venous serum concentrations of the drug (21-37% of those in maternal serum) closely paralleled those in the umbilical vein. Gentamicin was present in the fetal urine in concentrations 2-3 times those in the fetal serum, demonstrating the ability of the fetal kidneys to concentrate and excrete the drug. The drug was not detectable in the amniotic fluid, presumably due to the absence of fetal urination during the period of study. Daubenfeld et al. (1975) administered low (20 mg/hr) and high (40 mg/hr) doses of gentamicin to pregnant women during labor. Amniotic fluid levels of the drug rose at a slower rate than cord blood, but exceeded maternal serum concentrations after about 7 hours in the high dosage group.

Tobramycin traverses the placenta in a similar manner. Bernard et al. (1977) administered a single dose (2 mg/kg) of tobramycin intramuscularly to pregnant patients who were undergoing abortions during the first or second trimesters. Peak maternal serum levels of 4.0 μg/ml occurred after one hour. Tobramycin first appeared in fetal serum 2½ hours after maternal injection and this coincided with the highest concentration attained (0.58 μg/ml), which became undetectable by 17 hours. The highest and most persistent concentration was found in the fetal kidney, where tobramycin was demonstrable after two hours, and by nine hours, 53% of the fetal kidney samples had levels of 3 μg/gr or more. In the fetal urine, tobramycin was detected at 40 minutes, with the highest concentration (3.4 μg/ml) occurring after 2½ hours. Amniotic fluid levels appeared later and in pregnancies greater than 13 weeks, was first detected at 4 hours. Only 3 of 8 first trimester amniotic fluid samples (obtained at varying intervals post-drug administration) revealed tobramycin activity, whereas all of the second trimester samples had levels indicating a significant relationship with gestational age. In the cerebrospinal fluid, tobramycin was detected (but in low concentrations of 0.1-0.7 μg/ml) only in fetuses less than 17 weeks' gestation. The drug was not demonstrable in fetal lungs or livers.

Good and Johnson (1971) administered *kanamycin* (500 mg) intramuscularly to term pregnant women. Peak maternal (18.6 μg/ml) and cord (9.0 μg/ml) sera concentrations were reached after 60 and 135 minutes, respectively. The average level in cord serum was 6.0 μg/ml 3-6 hours following the injection, whereas in 6 hours, the mean level in amniotic fluid was 5.5 μg/ml.

At this time, we are unaware of any reports assessing the teratogenicity of gentamycin, tobramycin, and kanamycin; however, the available data are limited. A child with impaired hearing exposed in utero to kanamycin and ethacrynic acid at 28 weeks has been reported. The mother, who had renal impairment, developed ototoxicity while under treatment (Jones, 1973).

At present, one unresolved question is whether the fetus at different stages of gestation may be susceptible to toxic effects of the aminoglycosides at even lower concentrations than those producing damage in the adult.

Sulfonamides

This group of drugs appears to traverse the placenta with relative ease. Long-acting sulfonamides given to mothers during labor can be detected in cord blood and persist in the neonate several days after birth.

Sulfadimethoxine, a long-acting sulfonamide, administered orally during labor reaches maximal levels in the maternal blood 4-12 hours after ingestion. It has a half-life of 36 hours. The drug is demonstrable in the blood of the neonate during its first six days of life (Lucey and Driscoll, 1959). Since sulfonamides compete with bilirubin for albumin-binding and may cause or aggravate hyperbilirubinemia in the newborn, long-acting sulfonamides should be avoided when delivery is anticipated. A short-acting water soluble preparation should be chosen if a sulfonamide must be used during pregnancy. It should be mentioned that hyperbilirubinemia should not be a problem in the fetus since the placenta is capable of eliminating the bilirubin into the maternal blood.

Cotrimoxazole, a sulphamethoxazole-trimethoprim combination is sometimes used to treat urinary tract infection. One hundred and twenty pregnant patients (10 were less than 16 weeks) were given cotrimoxazole twice a day for seven days (Brumfitt and Pursell, 1973). In this study, no adverse fetal effects were noted. The number of patients studied, however, is relatively small to make a definitive statement about cotrimoxazole, particularly when used during the first trimester of pregnancy. It should be noted that trimethoprim is a powerful and selective inhibitor of dihydrofolate reductase, thereby blocking the synthesis of tetrahydrofolate. In view of this property, caution should be exercised meticulously in the use of this compound during pregnancy, particularly in the first trimester.

Tetracycline

Tetracyclines pose significant maternal and fetal risks so their use during pregnancy should be limited to those situations where no alternative therapy is available.

Larger doses of tetracycline may produce hepatic toxicity in pregnant and nonpregnant patients. Those with depressed liver or renal functions, as in pyelonephritis, are more prone to develop hepatotoxicity since the drug is primarily excreted by the kidney.

Tetracyclines cross the placenta with ease and rapidly reach the amniotic fluid. Leblanc and Perry (1967) administered 100 mg of tetracycline intravenously to 19 women in labor. They found that maternal serum levels fell rapidly from an average of 2.8 mcg/ml at 30 minutes to 1.0 mcg/ml and 0.2 mcg/ml at 4 and 9½ hours, respectively. Cord serum levels were 0.28 mcg/ml at 10 minutes, rose rapidly to an average of 1.5 mcg/ml at 1½ hours and fell to .1 mcg/ml at 9½ hours. The levels in cord serum were consistently lower than the corresponding maternal serum levels. The drug was detectable in the amniotic fluid within 19 minutes and reached .53 mcg/ml at 2.3 hours and .12 mcg/ml at 22½ hours.

Tetracycline deposits as a fluorescent compound primarily in calcifying teeth and bone. Calcification of the deciduous teeth of the fetus begins at about the end of the fourth month of gestation. Maternal intake of this drug during the second and third trimesters of pregnancy can therefore cause staining of the dentine and enamel. Genot and associates (1970) found no evidence that the affected teeth were predisposed to enamel hypoplasia or caries. Furthermore, no abnormalities of skeletal growth and general development were detected in 4-5-year-old children whose mothers had taken tetracycline during pregnancy.

The tetracycline-induced fluorescence can also be demonstrated in bones of neonates exposed prenatally to tetracycline. Such infants may show a transient inhibition of bone growth similar to that observed in premature infants given tetracycline (Cohlan, 1963). Whether an inhibition of growth in utero occurs in humans similar to that observed in animals is not entirely clear.

Apart from the preceding effects on bone and teeth, the degree, if any, of tetracycline teratogenicity in humans is unknown. An isolated case report of bilateral congenital deformities of the hand has been reported in an infant whose mother received tetracycline for 4 days at about 33 days of gestation. However, since the use of tetracycline during pregnancy is ill-advised, the question of teratogenicity in humans should be of limited practical value.

Chloramphenicol

Chloramphenicol is rapidly absorbed from the gastrointestinal tract reaching maximum blood levels in about two hours. Detoxification occurs in the liver predominantly by the action of glucuronyl transferase. Approximately 90% of a given dose is subsequently excreted by the kidney. The bulk of the excreted drug, which is an inactive glucuronide conjugate, is eliminated primarily by tubular secretion. Approximately 10% of the drug is excreted unaltered principally by glomerular filtration.

Chloramphenicol readily crosses the placenta in humans. Scott and Warner (1950) administered two grams of chloramphenicol orally to normal subjects who were at term and in labor. Therapeutic blood levels (6.3-39.8 μg/ml) were demonstrable within 71 minutes after a single dose and persisted for at least 135 minutes. The concentration of the drug in cord blood was comparable to that existing in the maternal circulation.

Fatal circulatory collapse (gray syndrome) in the newborn, especially the premature, has been attributed to chloramphenicol administration. The increased sensitivity in prematures may presumably be explained by the immaturity of the glucuronyl transferase system in the liver and decreased kidney function.

Retrospective studies have not implicated chloramphenicol as a possible teratogen (Nelson and Forfar, 1971; Heinonen et al., 1977). However, the possibility that chloramphenicol administered prior to delivery may induce gray syndrome in the neonate cannot be dismissed.

Chloramphenicol is not widely used in view of its potential hematologic toxicity. This should not be a deterrent factor in maternal life-threatening infections where other antibiotics are not efficacious.

Lincosamide Antibiotics

Lincomycin
Lincomycin traverses the placental barrier. Duignan et al. (1973) administered lincomycin intramuscularly (600 mg) to term pregnant patients. After a single dose, peak levels of 12.5 μg/ml were attained in maternal blood within 45 minutes. In cord blood, the highest levels (2.7 μg/ml) occurred after 55 minutes. Cord blood levels were generally 25% of corresponding maternal levels with both falling in a linear fashion. Levels less than 0.1 μg/ml were detected in maternal and cord blood 42 and 24 hours after injection. The concentrations attained in the amniotic fluid increased at a slower rate compared to the maternal and fetal blood but were higher than both after 16 hours.

A follow-up study of 92 children (age 7½ years) born to mothers given lincomycin at each trimester of pregnancy did not show any developmental anomaly or specific physical defects (Mickal and Panzer, 1975).

Clindamycin
Clindamycin is used in the treatment of documented anaerobic infections. In adults, pseudomembranous colitis may occur with its use; however, it is not known whether the fetus or the neonate can develop this problem when exposed in utero prior to delivery.

Clindamycin crosses the placenta readily. Weinstein et al. (1976) administered clindamycin (600 mg) intravenously to term pregnant patients. Maternal peak levels of 6-9 μg/ml were observed at the time of first sampling (15 minutes), falling gradually over the next 6-8 hours. The peak cord serum concentrations after 20 minutes were approximately 3 μg/ml which was 46% of levels present in maternal serum. The drug was not detectable in amniotic fluid during the first hour after injection. Philipson and co-workers (1973) administered a single oral dose (450 mg) to pregnant patients undergoing abortion in the first trimester. The average peak concentrations were 5.16 μg/ml and 0.32 μg/ml in maternal and cord sera, respectively. Amniotic fluid levels averaged .02 μg/ml. The drug was demonstrable in various fetal tissues—liver, kidney, spleen, lung, brain, and muscle—with the fetal liver concentration (0.4 to 1.8 μg/gram of tissue) exceeding levels present in fetal blood. The levels in various fetal organs were higher after maternal administration of multiple doses and within the accepted therapeutic range for the drug.

We are unaware of studies dealing with the embryotoxicity of clindamycin in humans.

Nitrofurantoin

Nitrofurantoin is commonly used in treating urinary tract infections. No untoward fetal effects have been reported with its use during pregnancy. A retrospective analysis of 101 patients with a maternal intake of 200-400 mg nitrofurantoin per day after the first trimester did not demonstrate any adverse effect upon apgar scores, evidence of jaundice or of congenital abnormalities (Perry et al., 1967a). However, hemolysis in the neonate can occur in the presence of G_6PD deficiency. Pulmonary hypersensitivity reaction has been described in the adult following the use of nitrofurantoin, including chronic interstitial pneumonitis and pulmonary fibrosis following prolonged use. It is unclear whether the fetus is susceptible to this hypersensitivity reaction.

Nitrofurantoin traverses the placenta rapidly and is detected in the cord and amniotic fluid at low concentrations for a short period, probably secondary to the drug's rapid half-life in the maternal circulation.

Perry infused nitrofurantoin to women in labor (1967b). Maternal serum levels determined immediately following the infusion ranged from 2.8-9.8 mcg/ml with a half-life of 32 ± 16 min. The cord levels 30 minutes after beginning the infusion were approximately 2.5 mcg/ml which became undetected after 1 hour. Amniotic fluid levels obtained at varying intervals (15 min to 20 hr) after the end of the infusion were very low and never exceeded 1.0 mcg/ml.

In the absence of available data, caution should be exercised in the use of nitrofurantoin for the treatment of urinary tract infections in the first trimester of pregnancy.

References and Recommended Reading

Barr, W, Graham, RM: Placental transmission of cephaloridine. J Obstet Gynaecol Br Commonw 74:739, 1967.

Bernard, B, Abate, M, Thielen, PF, Attar, H, Ballard, A, Wehrle, PF: Maternal-fetal pharmacological activity of amikacin. J Infect Dis 135:925, 1977.

Bernard, B, Barton, L, Abate, M, Ballard, CA: Maternal-fetal transfer of cefazolin in the first twenty weeks of pregnancy. J Infect Dis 136:377, 1977.

Bernard, B, Garcia, S, Ballard, CA, Ivler, D, Thruppe, L, Mathies, A, Wehrle, PF: Maternal-placental-fetal transfer of tobramycin. Clin Res 21:308, 1973.

Bernard, B, Garcia-Cazares, SJ, Ballard, CA, Thrupp, LD, Mathies, AW, Wehrle, PF: Tobramycin: Maternal-fetal pharmacology. Antimicrob Agents Chemother 11:688, 1977.

Belcher, TE, Edgar, WM, Melville, HAH, Peel, KR: Transplacental passage of ampicillin. Br Med J 1:137, 1966.

Bray, RE, Boe, RW, Johnson, WL: Transfer of ampicillin into fetus and amniotic fluid from maternal plasma in late pregnancy. Am J Obstet Gynecol 96:938, 1966.

Brumfitt, W, Pursell, R: Trimethoprim-sulfamethoxazole in the treatment of bacteriuria in women. J Infect Dis 128(Suppl):657S, 1973.

Burns, LE, Hodgman, JE, Cass, AB: Fatal circulatory collapse in premature infants receiving chloramphenicol. N Eng J Med 261:1318, 1959.

Carter, MP, Wilson, F: Antibiotics and congenital malformations. Lancet 1:1267, 1963. (Letter to the Editor)

Carter, MP, Wilson, F: Tetracycline and congenital limb abnormalities. Br Med J 2:407, 1962. (Letter to the Editor)

Cohlan, SQ: Tetracycline staining of teeth. Teratology 15:127, 1977.

Cohlan, SQ, Bevelander, G, Tiamsic, T: Growth inhibition of prematures receiving tetracycline. Am J Dis Child 105:453, 1963.

Conway, N, Birt, BD: Streptomycin in pregnancy: Effect on the foetal ear. Br Med J 2:260, 1965.

Corcoran, R, Castles, JM: Tetracycline for acne vulgaris and possible teratogenesis. Br Med J 2:807, 1977.

Daubenfeld, O, Modde, H, Hirsch, HA: Transfer of gentamicin to the foetus and the amniotic fluid during a steady state in the mother. (Abstract) Excerpta Medica (Ob/Gyn) 28:599, 1975.

Depp, R, Kind, AC, Kirby, WMM, Johnson, WL: Transplacental passage of methicillin and dicloxacillin into the fetus and amniotic fluid. Am J Obstet Gynecol 107:1054, 1970.

Duignan, NM, Andrews, J, Williams, JD: Pharmacological studies with lincomycin in late pregnancy. Br Med J 3:75, 1973.

Fenton, LJ, Light, IJ: Congenital syphilis after maternal treatment with erythromycin. Obstet Gynecol 47:492, 1976.

Genot, MT, Golan, HP, Porter, PJ, Kass, EH: Effect of administration of tetracycline in pregnancy on the primary dentition of the offspring. J Oral Med 25:77, 1970.

Glasko, AJ, Wolf, LM, Dill, WA, Bratton, Jr., C: Biochemical studies on chloramphenicol (Chloromycetin). J Pharmacol Exp Therap 96:445, 1949.

Good, RG, Johnson, GH: The placental transfer of kanamycin during late pregnancy. Obstet Gynecol 38:60, 1971.

Greene, GR: Tetracycline in pregnancy. N Eng J Med 295:512, 1976. (Letter to the Editor)

Harley, JD, Farrar, JF, Gray, JB, Dunlop, IC: Aromatic drugs and congenital cataracts. Lancet 1:472, 1964. (Preliminary communication)

Heinonen, OP, Slone, D, Shapiro, S: Antimicrobial and antiparasitic agents. In Heinonen, OP, Slone, D, Shapiro, S: Birth Defects and Drugs. Publishing Sciences Group, Inc., 1977, p. 296.

Hodgmann, JE, Burns, LE: Safe and effective chloramphenicol dosages for premature infants. Am J Dis Child 101:140, 1961.

Jones, HC: Intrauterine ototoxicity—A case report and review of the literature. J Nat Med Assoc 65:201, 1973.

Kauffman, RE, Morris, JA, Azarnoff, DL: Placental transfer and fetal urinary excretion of gentamicin during constant rate maternal infusion. Pediatr Res 9:104, 1975.

Kiefer, L, Rubin, A, McCoy, JB, Foltz, EL: The placental transfer of erythromycin. Am J Obstet Gynecol 69:174, 1955.

Kline, AH, Blattner, RJ, Lunin, M: Transplacental effect of tetracyclines on teeth. JAMA 188:178, 1964.

Kunin, CM: Clinical pharmacology of the new penicillins. I. The importance of serum protein binding in determining antimicrobial activity and concentration in serum. Clin Pharm Ther 7:166, 1966.

Leblanc, AL, Perry, JE: Transfer of tetracycline across the human placenta. Tex Rep Biol Med 25:541, 1967.

Lucey, JF, Driscoll, Jr., TJ: Hazard to newborn infants of administration of long-acting sulfonamides to pregnant women. Pediatrics 24:498, 1959. (Letter to the Editor)

Macaulay, JC, Leistyna, JA: Preliminary observations on the prenatal administration of demethylchlortetracycline HCl. Pediatrics 34:423, 1964.

MacAulay, MA, Abou-Sabe, M, Charles, D: Placental transfer of ampicillin. Am J Obstet Gynecol 96:943, 1966.

MacAulay, MA, Berg, SR, Charles, D: Placental transfer of dicloxacillin at term. Am J Obstet Gynecol 102:1162, 1968.

MacAulay, MA, Charles, D: Placental transfer of cephalothin. Am J Obstet Gynecol 100:940, 1968.

MacAulay, MA, Charles, D: Placental transmission of colistimethate. Clin Pharmacol and Therapeut 8:578, 1967.

MacAulay, MA, Molloy, WB, Charles, D: Placental transfer of methicillin. Am J Obstet Gynecol 115:58, 1973.

McCormack, WM, George, H, Donner, A, Kodgis, LF, Alpert, S, Lowe, EW, Dass, EH: Hepatotoxicity of erythromycin estolate during pregnancy. Antimicr Agent Chemother 12:630, 1977.

Mickal, A, Panzer, JD: The safety of lincomycin in pregnancy. Am J Obstet Gynecol 121:1071, 1975.

Morrow, S, Palmisano, P, Cassady, G: The placental transfer of cephalothin. J Pediatr 73:262, 1968.

Nelson, MM, Forfar, JO: Associations between drugs administered during pregnancy and congenital abnormalities of the fetus. Br Med J 1:523, 1971.

Nishimura, H, Tanimura, T: Chemotherapeutic Agents. In Nishimura, H, Tanimura, T: Clinical Aspects of the Teratogenicity of Drugs. Excerpta Medica, Amsterdam-Sidney, 1976, p. 121.

Perry, JE, Leblanc, AL: Transfer of ampicillin across the human placenta. Texas Rep Biol Med 25:547, 1967.

Perry, JE, Leblanc, AL: Transfer of nitrofurantoin across the human placenta. Texas Rep Biol Med 25:265, 1967(b).

Perry, JE, Toney, JD, Leblanc, AL: Effect of nitrofurantoin on the human fetus. Texas Rep Biol Med 25:270, 1967(a).

Persianinov, LS, Kirjushenkov, AN: Transplacental transport of antibiotics and their influence upon embryonic and fetal development. Excerpta Medica 412:110, 1977.

Philipson, A: Pharmacokinetics of ampicillin during pregnancy. J Infect Dis 136:370, 1977.

Philipson, A, Sabath, LD, Charles, D: Erythromycin and clindamycin absorption and elimination in pregnant women. Clin Pharm Ther 19:68, 1976.

Philipson, A, Sabath, LD, Charles, D: Transplacental passage of erythromycin and clindamycin. N Eng J Med 288:1219, 1973.

Prakash, A, Chalmers, JA, Onojobi, OIA, Henderson, RJ, Cummings, P: Transfer of limecycline and cephaloridine from mother to fetus—a comparative study. J Obstet Gynaecol Br Commonw 77:247, 1970.

Prochazka, J, Simkova, V, Havelka, J, Hejzlar, M, Viklicky, J, Kargerova, A, Kubikova, M: K otazce pruniku chloramfenikolu placentou. Cesk Pediatr (Praha) 19:311, 1964.

Rasmussen, F: The oto-toxic effect of streptomycin and dihydrostreptomycin on the foetus. Scand J Resp Dis 50:61, 1969.

Richards, IDG: Congenital malformations and environmental influences in pregnancy. Brit J Prev Soc Med 23:218, 1969.

Robinson, GC, Cambon, KG: Hearing loss in infants of tuberculous mothers treated with streptomycin during pregnancy. N Eng J Med 271:949, 1964.

Schardein, JL: Antimicrobial agents. In Drugs as Teratogens. CRC Press, Cleveland, Ohio, 1976, p. 155.

Scott, WC, Warner, RF: Placental transfer of chloramphenicol (chloromycetin). JAMA 142:1331, 1950.

Sutherland, JM: Fatal cardiovascular collapse of infants receiving large amounts of chloramphenicol. Am J Dis Child 97:761, 1959.

Totterman, LE, Saxen, L: Incorporation of tetracycline into human foetal bones after maternal drug administration. Acta Obstet Gynaecol Scand 48:542, 1969.

Tuchmann-Duplessis, H: Antimicrobial drugs. In Tuchmann-Duplessis, H, Drug Effects on the Fetus. Adis Press, Sydney, 1975, p. 128.

Udall, V: Toxicology of sulphonamidetrimethoprim combinations. Post Grad Med J 45(Suppl):42, 1969.

Varpela, E, Hietalahti, J, Aro, MJT: Streptomycin and dihydrostreptomycin medication during pregnancy and their effect on the child's inner ear. Scand J Resp Dis 50:101, 1969.

Wasz-Hockert, O, Nummi, S, Vuopala, S, Jarvinen, PA: Transplacental passage of azidocillin, ampicillin and penicillin G during early and late pregnancy. Scand J Infect Dis 2:125, 1970.

Weinstein, AJ, Gibbs, RS, Gallagher, M: Placental transfer of clindamycin and gentamicin in term pregnancy. Am J Obstet Gynecol 124:688, 1976.

Weiss, CF, Glazko, AJ, Weston, JK: Chloramphenicol in the newborn infant. N Eng J Med 262:787, 1960.

Westland, MM: Effects of tetracycline on chromosomes cultured from human lymphocytes. JAMWA 22:719, 1967.

Weyman, J: Tetracyclines and the teeth. Practitioner 195:661, 1965.

Williams, JD, Brumfitt, W, Codie, AP, Reeves, DS: The treatment of bacteriuria in pregnant women with sulphamethoxazole and trimethoprim. Post Grad Med J 45(Suppl):71, 1969.

Yoshioka, H, Monma, T, Matsuda, S: Placental transfer of gentamicin. Pediatr Pharmacol Therap 80:121, 1972.

ANTITUBERCULOSIS AGENTS

Lowe (1964) reported that the incidence of congenital defects among infants born to women under active treatment for pulmonary tuberculosis (including the first four months of pregnancy) is uncommon. In most instances, multiple drug therapy was used. This contrasted with an earlier study suggesting a significant association between congenital defects and a maternal history of tuberculosis (McDonald, 1961).

Currently, the most effective and well-tolerated drugs available for the treatment of tuberculosis are isoniazid, rifampin, ethambutol, and streptomycin. Secondary drugs include para-aminosalicylic acid, pyrazinamide, cycloserine, ethionamide.

There are a few clinical studies on the use of *ethambutol* during pregnancy. Reports dealing with a limited number of patients show no evidence of increased teratogenicity or impairment in fetal growth attributable to the drug (Bobrowitz, 1974; Lewitt et al., 1974). Postnatally, these children (aged 1 month to 9 years) showed normal growth and development (Bobrowitz, 1974). Because therapeutic doses can damage the optic nerve and eye tissue in sensitive patients, Lewitt et al. (1974) examined the embryos of six patients under ethambutol treatment who underwent elective abortions. Treatment was begun prior to conception and continued during the first twelve weeks of pregnancy. The total dosage was between 48-81 grams. The embryos did not show any gross malformations, and histologically the brain, nerves and sensory organs were normal. The authors point out, however, that functional impairment—especially of optic tissues—can only be detected on developmental follow-up.

The safety of *rifampin* during pregnancy has also not been established. Tuchmann-Duplessis cites the work of Jentgens (1973) in which 313 women received ethambutol and rifampin during pregnancy. Thirty-eight women took the medication prior to conception and during the first trimester. There was no drug-attributable embryotoxicity. Steen and Stainton-Ellis, in a letter to the Editor of *Lancet* (1977), report the finding of C. Pagani in which rifampin was used in 229 pregnancies. The incidence of malformations in this group was 4.3%. Pagani concluded that the risk of malformation was not high when compared with that of the disease itself and with the use of other antituberculosis therapy. A follow-up study on these children was not performed.

It is clear that additional studies are needed to fully evaluate the safety of rifampin and ethambutol during pregnancy.

References and Recommended Reading

Bobrowitz, ID: Ethambutol in pregnancy. Chest 66:20, 1974.

Citron, KM: Ethambutol: A review with special reference to ocular toxicity. Tubercle (Suppl):32, 1969.

Jentgens, H: Antituberkulase chemotherapie und Schwanger-Schaft-Sabbrunch. Prox Pneumologie 27:479, 1973.

Lewitt, T, Nebel, L, Terracina, S, Karman, S: Ethambutol in pregnancy: Observations on embryogenesis. Chest 66:25, 1974.

Lowe, CR: Congenital defects among children born to women under supervision or treatment for pulmonary tuberculosis. Br J Prev Soc Med 18:14, 1964.

McDonald, AD: Maternal health in early pregnancy and congenital defect. Final report on a prospective inquiry. Br J Prev Soc Med 15:154, 1961.

Steen, JSM, Stainton-Ellis, DM: Rifampicin in pregnancy. Lancet 2:604, 1977. (Letter to the Editor)

Tuchmann-Duplessis, H: Antimicrobial Drugs. In Tuchmann-Duplessis, H., Drug Effects on the Fetus, Adis Press, Sydney, 1975, p. 128.

ANTIDIABETICS

There is general agreement that the overall incidence of congenital malformations is increased in the offspring of pregnant diabetics. The exact cause of this increase is unknown, but it may relate to the severity of the diabetes and the adequacy of control. It is against this background that the possible embryotoxic effect of antidiabetic drugs has to be evaluated.

The traditional agent for treating diabetes mellitus is insulin. With the advent of the sulfonylureas, alternatives to insulin became available. These drugs have been used during pregnancy, but now are generally considered contraindicated in view of suspected embryotoxicity in the human, and the difficulty in achieving proper control in some patients. Currently, insulin remains the drug of choice during pregnancy, although the hormone has not escaped the teratogenic scrutiny.

Tolbutamide and Chlorpropamide

There is no proof that these drugs, in therapeutic doses, are teratogenic in the human; by the same token, we are unaware of studies that have specifically addressed themselves to this issue in order to reach a definite conclusion.

Dolger et al. (1962) reported favorably on 52 diabetic pregnancies treated with tolbutamide. Only one infant with major congenital malformation was recorded. Jackson and co-workers (1962) in a retrospective analysis compared pregnancy outcomes of chlorpropamide vs. tolbutamide-treated pregnancies. An excessive perinatal mortality was noted among the former but not the latter group. One infant of a tolbutamide-treated mother had severe malformations. This lack of an excess of congenital malformations among pregnant diabetics treated with sulfonylureas is also noted in various correspondence (Sterne, 1963; Malins et al., 1964). More recently Notelovitz (1971) reappraised the earlier data of Jackson et al. (1962) and reported on the pregnancy outcome of diabetics treated with tolbutamide (46 patients), chlorpropamide (58), and insulin (47). There were two newborn with obvious congenital malformations; one from a tolbutamide-treated mother, the other in a patient who received insulin after the 30th week. Contrary to earlier observations, an excess of perinatal mortality was not noted in properly controlled diabetics receiving the sulfonylureas. Chlorpropamide seemed a more effective agent than tolbutamide for the control of diabetes in pregnancy.

From their own experience and review of the literature, Sutherland and co-workers (1974) also found no evidence to support a direct effect of chlorpropamide in the formation of congenital malformations. The poor results in terms of perinatal morbidity and mortality could be explained by inadequate control of the diabetes rather than a specific fetal effect of the drug.

Both tolbutamide and chlorpropamide cross the placenta and can be detected in cord blood. A neonatal effect of these drugs should be watched for in mothers treated with sulfonylurea.

In summary, the balance of available evidence suggests that sulfonylureas are not teratogenic in humans, although as mentioned earlier, the evidence is not conclusive. Difficulties in proper diabetic control make these agents less than ideal for use during pregnancy, but it could be that in selected cases, and because of the advantage of their route of administration, sulfonylureas may have a role. It is not our purpose to discuss this aspect but only to point out that so far the problem with the use of these agents in pregnancy does not relate to an apparent teratogenic effect.

Insulin

Diabetes mellitus is associated with an overall increase in congenital malformations (predominantly in the cardiovascular and central nervous systems) and with the syndrome of phocomelic embryopathy. How much of this increase is inherent in the disease itself (i.e., the disturbance in carbohydrate metabolism) or in its treatment remains to be resolved. The latter touches upon the potential contribution to malformations made by hypo- or

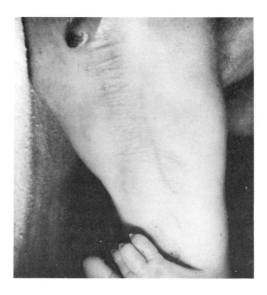

Fig. 3. Caudal regression syndrome. Infant born to a mother with diabetes mellitus.

hyper-glycemic states. Related or in addition to the issue of carbohydrate metabolism control is the question of insulin teratogenicity. This aspect has been discussed and reviewed by Assemany and co-workers (1972) and by Landauer (1972). Briefly, insulin is teratogenic when injected in chick and duck embryos and in various mammalian species when administered to the pregnant animal. The predominant anomalies relate to the skeletal system, which in some instances have a remarkable similarity to the phocomelic embryopathy associated with pregnancy in diabetic women. The mechanism(s) by which insulin induces the congenital anomalies could differ among the species studied but, at least in birds, seems not to be related to hypoglycemia but to be the outcome of a direct effect on the developing cells. Significantly, nicotinamide reduces the incidence of insulin-induced anomalies. Given in excess, however, nicotinamide itself becomes a teratogen.

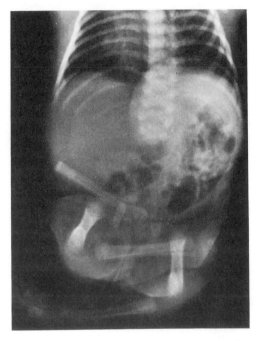

Fig. 4. X-ray film of another infant with caudal regression syndrome. Note that the spine is missing below L2. This infant was born to a mother with diabetes mellitus.

The possible contribution of insulin to the increased incidence of congenital malformations in diabetic women is a matter of conjecture. Maternally administered insulin does not cross the placenta, at least not in significant amounts. Furthermore, the higher rate of anomalies is also seen in non-insulin-requiring pregnant diabetics. Fetal hyperinsulinemia, on the other hand, may not account for all of the malformations noted for, according to Landauer, their occurrence precedes the state when the embryo produces insulin on its own. Be this as it may, the proper management of diabetes is the single most important factor in improving perinatal salvage— and the use of insulin is an integral part of that management.

70

References and Recommended Reading

Assemany, SR, Muzzo, S, Gardner, LI: Syndrome of phocomelic diabetic embryopathy (caudal dysplasia). Am J Dis Child 123:489, 1972.

Dolger, H, Bookman, JJ, Nechemias, C: The diagnostic and therapeutic value of tolbutamide in pregnant diabetics. Diabetes 11(Suppl):97, 1962.

Editorial: Abnormal infants of diabetic mothers. Lancet 1:633, 1980.

Jackson, WPU, Campbell, GD, Notelovitz, M, Blumsohn, D: Tolbutamide and chlorpropamide during pregnancy in human diabetics. Diabetes 11(Suppl):98, 1962.

Jervell, J, Bjerkedal, T, Moe, N: Outcome of pregnancies in diabetic mothers in Norway 1967-1976. Diabetologia 18:131, 1980.

Karlsson, K, Kjellmer, I: The outcome of diabetic pregnancies in relation to the mother's blood sugar level. Am J Obstet Gynecol 112:213, 1972.

Landauer, W: Is insulin a teratogen? Teratology 5:129, 1972.

Larsson, Y, Sterky, G: Possible teratogenic effect of tolbutamide in a pregnant prediabetic. Lancet 2:1424, 1960.

Malins, JM, Cooke, AM, Pyke, DA, Fitzgerald, MG: Sulphonylurea drugs in pregnancy. Br Med J 2:187, 1964. (Letter to the Editor)

Miller, DI, Wishinsky, H, Thompson, G: Transfer of tolbutamide across the human placenta. Diabetes 11(Suppl):93, 1962.

Notelovita, M: Oral hypoglycaemic therapy in diabetic pregnancies. Lancet 2:902, 1974. (Letter to the Editor)

Notelovitz, M: Sulphonylurea therapy in the treatment of the pregnant diabetic. S Afr Med J 45:226, 1971.

Rusnak, SL, Driscoll, SG: Congenital spinal anomalies in infants of diabetic mothers. Pediatrics 35:989, 1965.

Schiff, D, Aranda, JV, Stern, L: Neonatal thrombocytopenia and congenital malformations associated with administration of tolbutamide to the mother. J Pediatr 77:457, 1970.

Sobel, DE: Fetal damage due to ECT, insulin coma, chlorpromazine, or reserpine. AMA Arch Gen Psych 2:606, 1960.

Sterne, J: Antidiabetic drugs and teratogenicity. Lancet 1:165, 1963. (Letter to the Editor)

Sutherland, HW, Bewsher, PD, Cormack, JD, Hughes, CRT, Reid, A, Russell, G, Stowers, JM: Effect of moderate dosage of chlorpropamide in pregnancy on fetal outcome. Arch Dis Child 49:283, 1974.

Sutherland, HW, Stowers, JM, Cormack, JD, Bewsher, PD: Evaluation of chlorpropamide in chemical diabetes diagnosed during pregnancy. Br Med J 3:9, 1973.

ANTITHYROID DRUGS

The fetal thyroid is under pituitary control early in pregnancy, as evidenced by the presence of TSH in both the fetal pituitary gland and serum by the 8th-10th week of gestation. The synthesis of thyroid hormone by the fetal gland begins in the latter part of the first trimester. The fetal thyroid is able to concentrate iodine to a much larger extent than is the maternal thyroid.

Thioamide Compounds

Thioamide compounds (propylthiouracil and methimazole) and iodides are used in the treatment of thyrotoxicosis. These drugs cross the placenta and their administration during pregnancy has been associated with congenital goiter with or without fetal hypothyroidism. Larger goiters may cause mechanical dystocia during labor and delivery and cause airway obstruction after birth.

The administration of thioamide compounds has been associated with goiter in the fetus, presumably secondary to an increased fetal TSH secretion induced by the transplacental passage of the drugs. Histologically, the thyroid glands of fetuses exposed to propylthiouracil (PTU) have shown glandular hypertrophy and hyperplasia. Refetoff and co-workers (1974) described a transient neonatal hypothyroidism and/or goiter in two infants, each from a set of dizygotic twins, one of whose mothers received PTU and the other methimazole for the treatment of thyrotoxicosis. In both, serum TSH was elevated. One of the hypothyroid infants had a goiter which regressed spontaneously. In each set of twins, the other sibling was normal.

Neonatal goiter occurs only in a relatively small percentage of patients treated with thioamide drugs. In 26 pregnancies where either PTU or methimazole was used, 4 of the newborns had goiter. The reason for this relatively small incidence of congenital goiter is unclear, but does not seem to be dose-related. Burrow (1965) has suggested that the antithyroid medication may serve to manifest a mild inborn error in the synthesis of thyroid hormone by the fetus.

Iodides

Iodides decrease thyroid hormone production by blocking the organic binding of iodine. Although iodides are not recommended as primary agents in the management of hyperthyroidism during pregnancy, significant amounts of iodides can be ingested with the intake of iodide-containing cough preparations and expectorants.

Iodides taken by the pregnant woman during pregnancy can be goitrogenic to the fetus (Fig. 5). These goiters are generally larger than those associated with maternal intake of thiomides. Hypothyroidism, though sometimes of a transient nature, may be present in the neonate. The minimal dosage of elemental io-

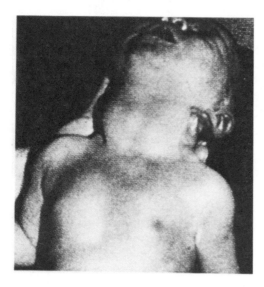

Fig. 5. Neonatal goiter associated with maternal iodide ingestion during pregnancy.

dine ingested by the mother that may induce fetal goiter has not been determined; however, Carswell and co-workers (1970) have reported two cases of congenital goiter in mothers whose intake of iodine was 12 mg/day. Unfortunately, the duration of therapy in these two patients was not specified. Similarly, the incidence of goiter in iodide-exposed fetuses cannot be gathered from the available data.

Another potential source of iodine are dyes used for contrast studies. Following the intraamniotic instillation of meglumine diatrizoate (for the purpose of amniography), levels of iodine in amniotic fluid have been found to be quite high as late as 24 hours after administration, becoming unmeasurable by 96 hours. Most of the measured iodine is, however, organically-bound and not free. No thyroid abnormalities were noted in the newborn; however, because of the small series, the authors could not exclude the possibility that meglumine diatrizoate used for amniography may cause fetal goiter.

In view of their goitrogenic effect and of the available alternative methods of treatment, iodides are not recommended for the treatment of thyrotoxicosis in pregnant women.

In addition to the effects on the fetal thyroid, congenital scalp defects have been associated with the intake of methimazole. This defect apart, there have been no other specific anomalies linked to the antithyroid drugs. In a series of 26 PTU or methimazole-exposed pregnancies (Mujtaba and Burrow, 1975), five infants had non-thyroid-related congenital defects. However, four of these were born to two mothers, raising the possibility of a genetic component. In their cumulative series of 68 patients, 9 infants were born with congenital abnormalities not related to the thyroid gland. Although this incidence is high, it is not possible to conclude from the available data that they were produced by the medications. Prospective studies with appropriate controls are needed to clarify this issue, and the degree, if any, of the teratogenicity of antithyroid medications remains an open question.

When thioamides are used, the minimum effective dose should be employed. At present, it appears that PTU is preferable to methimazole in view of the latter's incrimination in scalp defects. Neonates born to women taking antithyroid drugs should be considered at risk and thoroughly investigated for evidences of thyroid dysfunction. Necessary precautions should be made to cope with any respiratory obstructive problems in the neonate.

References and Recommended Reading

Anderson, GS, Bird, T: Congenital iodide goitre in twins. Lancet 2:742, 1961.

Ayromlooi, J: Congenital goiter due to maternal ingestion of iodides. Obstet Gynecol 39:818, 1972.

Bongiovanni, AM, Eberlein, WR, Thomas, PZ, Anderson, WB: Sporadic goiter of the newborn. J Clin Endocr 16:146, 1956.

Burrow, GN: Neonatal goiter after maternal propylthiouracil therapy. J Clin Endocr 25:403, 1965.

Burrow, GN, Bartsocas, C, Klatskin, EH, Grunt, JA: Children exposed in utero to propylthiouracil. Am J Dis Child 116:161, 1968.

Carswell, F, Kerr, MM, Hutchinson, JH: Congenital goitre and hypothyroidism produced by maternal ingestion of iodides. Lancet 1:1241, 1970.

Crepin, G, Delahousse, G, Decocq, J, et al.: Dangers des medicaments iodes chez la femme enceinte. Fraphlebologie 31:279, 1978. (Abstract in Excerpta Medica Sect Ob Gyn 36:397, 1979.)

Davis, LJ, Forbes, W: Thiouracil in pregnancy. Effect on fetal thyroid. Lancet 2:740, 1945.

73

ent of thyrotoxicosis with thiouracil. Lancet 1:171, 1945.

e management of thyroid disease in pregnancy. Postgrad

..cry, J: The physiology of thyroid function in pregnancy. Postgrad Med J 55:336, 1979.

Fisher, WD, Voorhess, ML, Gardner, LI: Congenital hypothyroidism in infant following maternal I therapy. J Pediatr 62:132, 1963.

Galina, MP, Avnet, NL, Einhorn, A: Iodides during pregnancy—An apparent cause of neonatal death. N Eng J Med 267:1124, 1962.

Hayashi, TT, Gilling, B: Placental transfer of thiouracil. Obstet Gynecol 30:736, 1967.

Iancu, T, Boyanower, Y, Laurian, N: Congenital goiter due to maternal ingestion of iodide. Am J Dis Child 128:528, 1974.

Milham, Jr., S, Elledge, W: Maternal methimazole and congenital defects in children. Teratology 5:125, 1972.

Morrison, JC, Boyd, M, Friedman, BI, Bucovaz, ET, Whybrew, WD, Koury, DN, Wiser, WL, Fish, SA: The effects of renografin-60 on the fetal thyroid. Obstet Gynecol 42:99, 1973.

Mujtaba, Q, Burrow, GN: Treatment of hyperthyroidism in pregnancy with propylthiouracil and methimazole. Obstet Gynecol 46:282, 1975.

Pharoah, POD, Buttfield, IH, Hetzel, BS: Neurological damage to the fetus resulting from severe iodine deficiency during pregnancy. Lancet 1:308, 1971.

Quinones, JD, Boyd, CM, Beierwaltes, WH, Poissant, GR: Transplacental transfer and tissue distribution of C-2-thiouracil in the fetus. J Nuc Med 13:148, 1972.

Raben, MS: Endocrine Conference. Arch Dis Child 13:469, 1953.

Refetoff, S, Ochi, Y, Selenkow, HA, Rosenfield, RL: Neonatal hypothyroidism and goiter in one infant of each of two sets of twins due to maternal therapy with antithyroid drugs. J Pediatr 85:240, 1974.

Saye, EB, Watt, CH, Foushee, JC, Palmar, JI: Congenital thyroid hyperplasia in twins. JAMA 149:1399, 1952.

Senior, B, Chernoff, HL: Iodide goiter in the newborn. Pediatrics 47:510, 1971.

Serup, J: Fetal and neonatal hypothyroidism due to antithyroid-drug therapy. Lancet 2:845, 1978. (Letter)

Wolff, J: Iodide goiter and the pharmacologic effects of excess iodide. Am J Med 47:101, 1969.

METHYLXANTHINES
Caffeine
Caffeine is one of the most, if not the most, commonly ingested drug among a large segment of the world population. It is present in significant amounts in coffee, tea, colas, chocolate, and in many of the over-the-counter medications used for headaches and upper respiratory tract infections. A high percentage of pregnant women ingest one or more of these products. Caffeine readily crosses the placenta, and its level in first trimester fetal tissues is similar to that in maternal plasma.

In pregnant animals caffeine is found in uterine secretions approaching concentrations higher than those found in the maternal plasma. Caffeine is also present in human fetal cord blood and in the amniotic fluid. In nonpregnant subjects the half-life of caffeine in the serum varies between 2-6 hours.

Certain presumed effects of caffeine raise concern for its potential fetal effects. The mutagenic and carcinogenic properties of caffeine have not been resolved even experimentally. In very high doses caffeine is teratogenic in experimental animals, whereas in lower doses (higher on a weight basis than most daily caffeine consumption by humans), the findings are not striking. Epidemiologic surveys seem to indicate a higher incidence of pregnancy wastage among men or women with an estimated daily caffeine intake of 400 mg or over (roughly equivalent to 5-7 servings of non-decaffeinated coffee, 12-15 of tea, and 9-10 of cola per day). These surveys do not necessarily establish a cause-effect relationship. Multifactorial interactions have not been analyzed sufficiently to make a definitive statement possible. At this time, however, it seems prudent to advise women against excessive caffeine intake during pregnancy.

Theophylline

Theophylline, another methylxanthine, is used in the treatment of asthma. Theophylline has a wide range of pharmacologic effects. Its exact mechanism of action has not been fully worked out, although it seems to relate to inhibition of cyclic nucleotide phosphodiesterases. Theophylline is absorbed from the stomach and small intestines, and more uniformly when given by retention enema. It is weakly ionized in maternal plasma and hence crosses the placental "barrier" easily. Its concentration in cord blood at delivery is similar to that of maternal plasma. Compared to the adult, the neonate eliminates theophylline slowly, its half-life being 2-3 times that in adults. This decreased metabolism is probably due to deficiency of the cytochrome P450 monoxygenase system which N- demethylates the drug. Premature newborn may transform theophylline into caffeine, a reaction that does not occur in adults; the latter drug can then exert its own effects. Fetal livers from 12-20-week abortuses methylate theophylline into caffeine which appears to be the principal metabolite.

There is a dearth of information on the issue of theophylline teratogenicity. Findings compatible with theophylline toxicity such as jitteriness, irritability, tachycardia, gagging and vomit-

76

ing, have occurred in offspring of theophylline-treated mothers, despite a cord blood level of the drug below the generally accepted limits for toxicity in adults. This, at least in part, may be due to the lowered binding of the drug in the newborn blood increasing the relative concentration of the free moiety. Because of this potential, signs of theophylline toxicity should be looked for in infants of theophylline-exposed mothers.

As of the present, we are unaware of a presumed teratogenic effect of theophylline in man; in view of the maternal fetal risk of uncontrolled asthma, theophylline treatment would be indicated where warranted. Theophylline may even be of benefit in the treatment of apnea in premature babies.

References and Recommended Reading

Aranda, JV, Louridas, AT, Vitullo, BB, Thom, P, Aldridge, A, Haber, R: Metabolism of theophylline to caffeine in human fetal liver. Science 206:1319, 1979.

Aranda, JV, Sitar, DS, Parsons, WD, et al.: Pharmacokinetic aspects of theophylline in premature newborns. N Engl J Med 295:413, 1976.

Arwood, LL, Dasta, JF, Friedman, C: Placental transfer of theophylline: Two case reports. Pediatrics 63:844, 1979.

Barrett, CT, Sevanian, A, Lavin, N, et al: Role of adenosine 3'.5'-monophosphate in maturation of fetal lungs. Pediatr Res 10:621, 1976.

Blake, RL: Caffeine: Its effect on pregnancy. Post Grad Med 63:48, 1978.

Bory, C, Baltassat, P, Porthault, M, et al.: Biotransformation of theophylline to caffeine in premature newborn. Lancet 2:1204, 1978.

Gilbert, RM, Marshman, JA, Schwieder, M, et al.: Caffeine content of beverages as consumed. Canada Med Assoc J 114:205, 1976.

Goldstein, A, Warren, R: Passage of caffeine into human gonadal and fetal tissue. Biochem Pharmacol 17:166, 1962.

Hill, RM: Drugs ingested by pregnant women. Clin Pharmacol Ther 14:654, 1973.

Kang, ES: Cyclic nucleotide phosphodiesterase activities of the fetal and mature human cerebral cortex. Pediatr Res 11:655, 1977.

Karotkin, EH, Kido, M, Cashore, WJ, et al.: Acceleration of fetal lung maturation by aminophylline in pregnant rabbits. Pediatr Res 10:722, 1976.

Mulvihill, J: Caffeine as teratogen and mutagen. Teratology 8:69, 1973.

Palm, PE, Arnold, EP, Rachwall, PC, Leyczek, JC, Teague, KW, Kensler, CJ: Evaluation of the teratogenic potential of fresh-brewed coffee and caffeine in the rat. Toxicol Appl Pharmacol 44:1, 1978.

Parsons, WD, Aranda, JV, Neims, AH: Elimination of transplacentally acquired caffeine in full-term neonates. Pediatr Res 10:333, 1976.

Sieber, SM, Fabro, S: Identification of drugs in the preimplantation blastocyte and in the plasma, uterine secretion and urine of the pregnant rabbit. J Pharmacol Exp Ther 176:65, 1971.

Smyly, DS, Woodward, BB, Conrad, EC: Determination of saccharin, sodium benzoate and caffeine in beverages by reverse phase high pressure liquid chromatography. J Assoc Anal Chem 59:14, 1976.

Sommer, KR, Hill, RM, Horning, MG: Identification and quantification of drugs in human amniotic fluid. Res Commun Chem Pathol Pharmacol 12:583, 1975.

Thayer, P, Palm, P: A current assessment of mutagenic and teratogenic effects of caffeine. CRC Crit Rev Toxicol 5:345, 1975.

Timson, J: Caffeine. Mutation Res 47:1, 1977.

Weathersbee, PS, Lodge, JR: Caffeine: Its direct and indirect influence on reproduction. J Reprod Med 19:55, 1977.

Weathersbee, PS, Olsen, LK, Lodge, JR: Caffeine and pregnancy—A retrospective survey. Post Grad Med 62:64, 1977.

Yeh, TF, Pildes, RS: Transplacental aminophylline toxicity in a neonate. Lancet 1:910, 1977.

BROMOCRIPTINE AND CLOMIPHENE

Bromocriptine

Bromocriptine, 2 bromo α ergocryptine, is an ergot derivative that inhibits the secretion of prolactin (PRL) in man and other species. It is rapidly and efficiently absorbed from the gastrointestinal tract. It is extensively metabolized in the body, the principal excretory pathway being the biliary system and to a lesser extent the kidney. It acts both on the pituitary and hypothalamus. The duration of action is up to eight hours and is dependent on the dose and prolactin levels. Bromocriptine has less specific effects on hormones other than prolactin secretion. Gastrointestinal, cardiovascular and both central and peripheral nervous system effects have been described.

Clinically, bromocriptine has been employed in the management of a variety of conditions. Its main use, however, is in the treatment of hyperprolactinemia, frequently manifested in the galactorrhea-amenorrhea syndromes. As a sequela to treatment, ovulation and hence conception may occur. Since the accompanying disease, e.g., pituitary adenoma, may necessitate the maintenance of therapy during pregnancy, the effect of the drug on pregnancy outcome assumes clinical relevance.

The experience with bromocriptine administered during pregnancy is admittedly limited. However, because of current awareness of the importance of evaluating drug safety during pregnancy, the experience with bromocriptine is becoming fairly well documented. In rats, rabbits, and primates bromocriptine in doses (mg/kg) higher than those used therapeutically in humans appears to be non-teratogenic; cleft palate has been infrequently and inconsistently noted in certain rabbit strains, but a cause-effect relationship is at best uncertain.

The experience with bromocriptine and pregnancy in the human may be divided into two groups: those in whom bromocriptine was discontinued soon after conception, and those in whom the drug was continued throughout pregnancy.

Bromocriptine Exposure in Early Pregnancy

Thomas et al. (1977) reported on 13 women with hyperprolactinemia treated with bromocriptine in whom the drug was discontinued four days after the expected date of a menstrual period. The pregnancies continued to term and fetal and placental weights were normal. The sex ratio of the offspring was similar to controls. Prolactin levels in the first trimester tended to be higher than in the controls. Serum progesterone levels were lower in the 11-12-week interval, but did not differ from controls thereafter. Essentially similar results were reported by Pepperell et al. (1977). Others, including case studies only, have also reported on fetal outcome in hyper- and normal prolactinemic patients, with or without pituitary tumors, in whom bromocriptine was discontinued at the earliest indication of pregnancy (from 2-21 days after expected date of menstruation) (Thorner et al., 1975; Mornex et al., 1978; Bergh et al., 1978; Moggi et al., 1979; Cowden and Thomson, 1979; Isaacs, 1979; Shewchuk et al., 1980; Griffith et al., 1979).

Thus the cumulative experience to date shows that pregnancies following bromocriptine-induced ovulation—where the drug is discontinued soon after conception—are not associated with an increase in either overall or specific incidence of congenital malformations.

Bromocriptine throughout Pregnancy

Although in most instances bromocriptine therapy may be discontinued once pregnancy is achieved, potential need for it during pregnancy may arise. This applies particularly to pregnancies in women with PRL producing micro- or macroadenomas of the pituitary. The efficacy of the ergot derivative in the management of these patients—especially those with microadenomas—is being investigated, predominantly in nonpregnant subjects, with promising results.

From their survey Gemzell and Wang (1979) concluded that

during pregnancy, the risk of complications relating to pituitary adenomas correlated with their size and treatment. The incidence of complications for untreated micro- and macroadenomas was 5.5 and 35.7%, respectively, and for treated adenomas, 7.1%. Complications such as visual field disturbances arising during pregnancy necessitate therapy. Gemzell and Wang have recommended that should visual field defects develop during pregnancy in patients with prolactin-producing microadenomas, bromocriptine therapy be employed, and that in patients with PRL-producing macroadenomas who develop visual field defects, bromocriptine be the treatment of choice. The authors mention a pregnant patient who developed visual field defects at 30 weeks and was successfully treated with bromocriptine resulting in a term delivery. Unfortunately, the duration of therapy and other pertinent details are not provided.

To date the use of bromocriptine during pregnancy has been limited. Concern regarding potential teratogenic and oxytocic properties are contributing factors. As indicated earlier, animal experiments have not established that the ergot derivative is teratogenic, and in rabbits it demonstrates no oxytocic properties on the smooth muscle of the uterus (Strumer and Fluckiger, 1974, cited by Mehta and Tolis, 1979). Despite these assurances from animal investigations, experience in humans is still needed to evaluate the safety of the drug during human pregnancy.

Del-Pozo and co-workers (1977) reported on one patient treated with bromocriptine (5 mg per day) throughout pregnancy because of symptomatic mammary hypertrophy. Details of the progress of the pregnancy are not provided. Delivery occurred at 38 weeks, resulting in an apparently healthy infant of normal birth weight. The course of pregnancy in an acromegalic woman treated with 10 mg of bromocriptine throughout pregnancy was reported by Bigazzi et al. in 1979. The pregnancy progressed normally and a healthy male infant was born whose development was followed up to 1½ years of age. Both somatic and psychic growth were normal.

In a letter to the Editor of *Lancet*, Yuen (1978) described two patients with prolactin-secreting microadenomas of the pituitary treated with bromocriptine into the third trimester of pregnancy. Both pregnancies resulted in healthy infants at term (one male, one female) of normal birth weights. One patient received 2.5-7.5 mg bromocriptine daily up to the 35th week; the other 2.5-5 mg daily up to 33 weeks. In another letter to the Editor of *Lancet*, Espersen and Ditzel (1977) mention the pregnancy outcome in an acromegalic woman with galactorrhea who received 35 mg of bromocriptine daily during her pregnancy. The patient went into labor at 33 weeks following spontaneous rupture of the membranes. A healthy 1580-gram infant was born who developed normally.

Effect of Bromocriptine on the Endocrine System During Pregnancy—Studies in Sheep

Martal and Lacroix (1978) studied the effect of bromocriptine (1 mg s.c. 2X 1 day) in pregnant ewes beginning on day 70 of gestation. The concentration of ovine chorionic somatomammotropin in the placenta peaked around 100 days of gestation, becoming 4-6 times higher than the level in placentas of nontreated ewes. The concentration thereafter fell and became similar in the two groups. Significantly, the peak placental concentration of the chorionic somatomammotropin in the control ewes was reached between 110-120 days. Thus bromocriptine not only increased the concentration of the hormone but advanced the timing of its peak levels in the placenta. Contrary to the findings in the placenta, the maternal and fetal serum concentrations of chorionic somatomammotropin were not altered by bromocriptine treatment. As anticipated, PRL levels in the sera of the bromocriptine-treated ewes were significantly reduced, but the levels in the fetal sera were unchanged. A significant reduction in the weight of corpora lutea up to 120 days was noted with bromocriptine treatment. No differences were noted in the fetal and placental weights.

Bromocriptine infusion into the pregnant ewe or her fetus lowers their respective plasma prolactin levels (Lowe et al., 1979). It also depresses ovine chorionic somatomammotropin in maternal but not in fetal plasma, and does not affect the duration of gestation.

Human Studies

The work of Del-Pozo et al. (1977) and Bigazzi et al. (1979) shed some light on the influence of bromocriptine on the endocrine system during pregnancy. In the patient reported by Del-Pozo and associates, the mean PRL level in maternal blood throughout the pregnancy was decreased. Amniotic fluid PRL concentrations, however, were within normalcy, as was the level in the newborn. The maternal and newborn plasma concentrations of placental lactogen were not altered. In the case reported by Bigazzi et al., bromocriptine given for the duration of pregnancy showed no influence on maternal plasma estradiol, estriol, or progesterone levels or on 24-hour urinary estriol excretion. As in previous findings, maternal plasma PRL concentrations were suppressed as was the level in the infant's plasma; prolactin levels in the amniotic fluid were normal; and the placental lactogen levels in the maternal blood were unaltered.

Summary
The experience to date with bromocriptine and pregnancy shows that when the drug is discontinued up to three weeks after conception no harmful effects of the drug on the fetus have been observed; hence, a normal pregnancy outcome can be anticipated. The documented experience with pregnancy outcome when the drug is taken throughout pregnancy is severely limited, however, and consists predominantly of case reports. Nevertheless, the evidence such as it is does not point to any adverse effects on the fetus. This should make it possible, within a strictly controlled framework, to administer the drug for valid indications during pregnancy, where the benefits clearly outweigh the possible risks involved.

Clomiphene
Clomiphene is a triphenylethylene derivative which is used clinically to induce ovulation. The likelihood of its producing multiple gestation is well established. Concern has been raised about the potential teratogenicity of clomiphene in the human. While no final conclusion can be reached, the balance of evidence seems to favor a lack of—or at worst a low degree of—teratogenicity. The widely differing findings addressing themselves to this issue may be at least partly explained by some of the drawbacks of case reporting and epidemiologic survey. It should be mentioned that the outcome of clomiphene-induced pregnancies should properly be compared to that of subfertile appropriately matched subjects, and not to that of normal fertile women. Viewed from this perspective, it is difficult to show that clomiphene-induced pregnancies have a higher rate of pregnancy wastage or congenital malformations at term, nor do the findings appear to differ from those of gonadotropin-induced pregnancies. The dosage of clomiphene and the number of treatment cycles do not seem to influence the pregnancy outcome.

The preceding remarks refer to clomiphene-induced pregnancies, and do not take into account inadvertent clomiphene exposure after conception has occurred. This aspect is avoidable and hence should not be of major concern.

References and Recommended Reading

Adashi, EY, Rock, JA, Sapp, KC, Martin, EJ, Wentz, AC, Jones, GS: Gestational outcome of clomiphene-related conceptions. Fertil Steril 31:620, 1979.

Ahlgren, M, Kallen, B, Rannevik, G: Outcome of pregnancy after clomiphene therapy. Acta Obstet Gynecol Scand 55:371, 1976.

Bergh, T, Nillius, SJ, Wide, L: Clinical course and outcome of pregnancies in amenorrhoeic women with hyperprolactinaemia and pituitary tumours. Br Med J 1:875, 1978.

Bigazzi, M, Ronga, R, Lancranjan, I, et al.: A pregnancy in an acromegalic woman during bromocriptine treatment: Effects on growth hormone and prolactin in the maternal, fetal, and amniotic compartments. J Clin Endocr Metab 48:9, 1979.

Clemens, MR, Goeser, R, Keller, E, et al.: Intrauterine development, feto-placental function and pregnancy outcome after induction of ovulation with bromoergocryptine. Excerpta Medica Ob Gyn 35:143, 1979.

Cowden, EA, Thomson, JA: Resolution of hyperprolactinaemia after bromocriptine-induced pregnancy. Lancet 1:613, 1979. (Letter to the Editor)

Del-Pozo, E, Darragh, A, Lancranjan, I, et al.: Effect of bromocriptin on the endocrine system and fetal development. Clin Endocrinol 6:47S, 1977.

Espersen, T, Ditzel, J: Pregnancy and delivery under bromocriptine therapy. Lancet 2:985, 1977. (Letter to the Editor)

Gemzell, C, Wang, CF: Outcome of pregnancy in women with pituitary adenoma. Fertil Steril 31:363, 1979.

Griffith, RW, Turkalj, I, Braun, P: Outcome of pregnancy in mothers given bromocriptine. Br J Clin Pharmacol 5:227, 1978.

Griffith, RW, Turkalj, I, Braun, P: Pituitary tumours during pregnancy in mothers treated with bromocriptine. Br J Clin Pharmacol 7:393, 1979.

Human Pituitary Advisory Committee, Australian Health Department, Canberra: Birth weight in pregnancies after induction of ovulation with pituitary gonadotrophins. Med J Aust 2:549, 1975.

Isaacs, AJ: Resolution of hyperprolactinaemia after bromocriptine-induced pregnancy. Lancet 1:784, 1979. (Letter to the Editor)

Jurgensen, O, Taubert, HD: Cervical incompetence and premature delivery after bromocriptine therapy for fertility. Lancet 2:203, 1977. (Letter to the Editor)

Lamberts, SWJ, Klijn, JGM, deLange, SA, Singh, R, Stefanko, SZ, Birkenhager, JC: The incidence of complications during pregnancy after treatment of hyperprolactinemia with bromocriptine in patients with radiologically evident pituitary tumors. Fertil Steril 31:614, 1979.

Lowe, KC, Beck, NF, McNaughton, DC, et al.: Effect of long-term bromocriptine infusion on plasma prolactin and ovine chorionic somatomammotropin in the pregnant ewe and fetal sheep. Am J Obstet Gynecol 135:773, 1979.

Mainoya, JR: Possible influence of prolactin on intestinal hypertrophy in pregnant and lactating rats. Experimentia 34:1230, 1978.

Martal, J, Lacroix, MC: Production of chorionic somatomammotropin (oCS), fetal growth of the placenta and the corpus luteum in ewes treated with 2-bromo-α-ergocryptine. Endocrinology 103:193, 1978.

Mehta, AE, Tolis, G: Pharmacology of bromocriptine in health and disease. Drugs 17:313, 1979.

Modena, G, Portioli, I: Delivery after bromocriptine therapy. (Letter) Lancet 2:558, 1977.

Moggi, G, Giampietro, O, Chisci, R, Brunori, I, Simonini, N: Pregnancy induction after bromocriptine-cyclofenil treatment in some normoprolactinemic anovulatory women. Fertil Steril 32:289, 1979.

Mornex, R, Orgiazzi, J, Hugues, B, Gagnaire, JC, Claustrat, B: Normal pregnancies after treatment of hyperprolactinemia with bromoergocryptine, despite suspected pituitary tumors. J Clin Endocr Metab 47:290, 1978.

Oakley, GP, Flynt, JW: Increased prevalence of Down's syndrome (mongolism) among the offspring of women treated with ovulation-inducing agents. Teratology 5:264, 1972.

Pepperell, RJ, McBain, JC, Winstone, SM, Smith, MA, Brown, JB: Corpus luteum function in early pregnancy following ovulation induction with bromocriptine. Br J Obstet Gynaecol 84:898, 1977.

Shewchuk, AB, Adamson, GD, Lessard, P, Ezrin, C: The effect of pregnancy on suspected pituitary adenomas after conservative management of ovulation defects associated with galactorrhea. Am J Obstet Gynecol 136:659, 1980.

Strumer, E, Fluckiger, E: In vivo smooth muscle stimulant activity of 2-Br-α-ergocryptine as compared with that of ergotamine. IRCS Med Sci Library Compendium 2:1591, 1974.

Thomas, CMG, Corbey, RS, Rolland, R: Assessment of unconjugated oestradiol and progesterone serum levels throughout pregnancy in normal women and in women with hyperprolactinaemia, who conceived after bromocriptine treatment. Acta Endocrinologica 86:405, 1977.

Thorner, MO, Besser, GM, Jones, A, Dacie, J, Jones, AE: Bromocriptine treatment of female infertility: Report of 13 pregnancies. Br Med J 4:694, 1975.

Yuen, BH: Bromocriptine, pituitary tumours, and pregnancy. Lancet 2:1314, 1978. (Letter to the Editor)

Ziegler, MG, Lake, CR, Williams, AC, et al.: Bromocriptine inhibits norepinephrine release. Clin Pharmacol Therap 25:137, 1979.

ANTIHISTAMINES

Probably the most frequent use of drugs in this category during pregnancy has been for the treatment of "morning sickness." Following the suggestion that these drugs may be teratogenic to the human fetus, their use during pregnancy has been markedly decreased if not discontinued by many physicians.

The evidence that meclizine hydrochloride and pyridoxine hydrochloride, singly or in combination, are teratogenic in humans is far from conclusive. The initial suggestions did not emanate from well-controlled studies, and several subsequent reports have not confirmed a teratogenic effect (Watson, 1962;

Leck, 1962; James, 1963; McBride, 1963). A prospective study by Smithells and Chinn (1964) produced no evidence supporting the teratogenicity of meclizine in the human. Yerushalmy and Milkovich (1965) in an extensive analysis evaluated the question of teratogenicity of the meclizine drugs in humans. They concluded, with "reasonable assurance," that these drugs were not teratogenic when used in conventional dosage. Indeed one might say that a possible beneficial effect in subjects may occasionally be gleaned when compared to those with untreated morning sickness. Nevertheless, these and similar drugs should not and need not be routinely prescribed. It is our impression that their true indication arises quite infrequently.

The recommendations to the Food and Drug Administration by the Ad Hoc Advisory Committee on the Teratogenic Effect of Certain Drugs regarding cyclizine, chlorcyclizine and meclizine, and the actions taken by the Food and Drug Administration are reported by Sadusk and Palmisano (1965).

There is less direct information on the fetal safety of other antihistamines. In a retrospective study, Nelson and Forfar (1971) found no association between congenital malformations and the intake of antihistamines during the first trimester of pregnancy. The drugs included promethazine hydrochloride, diphenhydramine, mepyramine maleate, chlorpheniramine, and diphenylpyraline, among others. Similarly, in their comprehensive and detailed analysis, Heinonen and co-workers (1977) did not find an association between exposure to antihistamines during the first-to-fourth lunar months and uniform malformations.

A possible link between diphenhydramine and cleft palate has been suggested, but needs confirmation (Saxen, 1974). Furthermore, tremulousness and diarrhea have been observed on the 5th day of life in a newborn where the blood level of the drug was 0.7 mg/ml. The mother had received 150 mg daily of diphenhydramine during her pregnancy (duration of therapy not specified). These symptoms were interpreted as representing withdrawal rather than toxic manifestations (Parkin and Bliss, 1974). Despite the tenuousness of these observations, pregnant women should be made aware of these possibilities.

The need for antihistamines may arise during pregnancy in patients with asthma. As with all other medications, the benefit-risk evaluation has to be frankly and comprehensively discussed with the patient. It is heartening, however, to realize that the evidence to date does not indict many of the antihistamines as being teratogenic. Several of these drugs appear to be reasonably safe during pregnancy.

References and Recommended Reading

David, A, Goodspeed, AH: "Ancoloxin" and foetal abnormalities. (Letter) Br Med J 1:121, 1963.

Greenberger, P, Patterson, R: Safety of therapy for allergic symptoms during pregnancy. Ann Int Med 89:234, 1978.

Heinonen, OP, Slone, D, Shapiro, S: Birth defects and drugs in pregnancy. Littleton, Mass, Publ Sciences Group, 1977, p. 322.

Idanpaan-Heikkila, J, Saxen, L: Possible teratogenicity of imipramine/chloropyramine. Lancet 2:282, 1973.

James, JR: "Ancoloxin" and foetal abnormalities. (Letter) Br Med J 1:59, 1963.

Leck, IM: Letter ("Ancoloxin") Br Med J 2:1610, 1962.

Lenz, W: Malformations caused by drugs in pregnancy. Am J Dis Child 112:99, 1966.

Martin-Nahon, L: "Ancoloxin" and foetal abnormalities. (Letter) Br Med J 1:331, 1963.

McBride, WG: An aetiological study of drug ingestion by women who gave birth to babies with cleft palates. Aust New Zeal J Obstet Gynaecol 9:103, 1969.

McBride, W: Cyclizine and congenital abnormalities. (Letter) Br Med J 1:1157, 1963.

Nelson, MM, Forfar, JO: Association between drugs administered during pregnancy and congenital abnormalities of the fetus. Br Med J 1:523, 1971.

Parkin, DE, Bliss, RW: Probable Benadryl withdrawal manifestations in a newborn infant. (Letter) J Pediatr 85:580, 1974.

Sadusk, JF, Palmisano, PA: Teratogenic effect of meclizine, cyclizine, and chlorcyclizine. JAMA 194:987, 1965.

Saxen, I: Cleft palate and maternal diphenhydramine intake. (Letter) Lancet 1:407, 1974.

Slone, D, Shapiro, S: Drugs and pregnancy. (Letter) Ann Int Med 90:275, 1979.

Smithells, RW, Chinn, ER: Meclozine and foetal malformations: A prospective study. Br Med J 1:217, 1964.

Watson, GI: Meclozine ("Ancoloxin") and foetal abnormalities. Br Med J 2:1446, 1962.

Yerushalmy, J, Milkovich, L: Evaluation of the teratogenic effect of meclizine in man. Am J Obstet Gynecol 93:553, 1965.

OTHER DRUGS

Aspirin

Compared with the widespread use of salicylates, there is relatively little information on the teratogenicity of salicylates in the human. In high doses salicylates are clearly teratogenic in various species including monkeys where the teratogenic dose is several times larger than that needed in rats. This may be at least partly explained by the differing pharmacodynamics of aspirin in these species. The embryotoxicity of salicylates—which is not uniform among the various species—includes growth retardation, rib malformations, cleft lips, and other cranial anomalies as well as constrictions of the ductus arteriosus. Significantly, the embryotoxic effects of salicylates can be enhanced by other environmental factors such as malnutrition, maternal stress, and benzoic acid. These observations may have relevance to the situation in man, in that although per unit weight human consumption of salicylates is below that used in the animal studies, the potentiation of salicylate toxicity by other factors may render otherwise innocuous levels harmful. This aspect, as with other drugs, warrants closer scrutiny.

The available data in humans are less precise and often conflicting. This is partly due to the nature of the studies, mainly retrospective, to the differing methods of selecting the study population, and to the failure to allow for the multifarious influences that could affect the outcome.

Perhaps the difficulty in arriving at a firm conclusion on the question of fetal effects of aspirin in the human may be illustrated by examining two reports appearing within one year of each other in the same journal. In 1975, Turner and Collins in Australia reported on the outcome in newborns of 144 mothers who took salicylates regularly during their pregnancy. Previous reports had raised the suspicion of aspirin teratogenicity in humans by finding that a higher proportion of mothers of babies with anomalies had taken salicylates than had mothers of controls. Turner and Collins assayed salicylate levels in maternal and cord blood at delivery. Their study failed to demonstrate an increased incidence of malformations, although there was an association with fetal growth retardation and increased perinatal mortality. The decrease in birth weight seemed more pronounced the longer salicylates were ingested. Elevated levels of salicylates in cord blood were not associated with apparent clinical abnormalities, nor was the higher perinatal mortality fully explained by antepartum hemorrhage, postdatism, or low birth weight.

Shapiro et al. in the United States reported on a cohort study of 41,337 gravidas from a collaborative perinatal project, of whom 26,381 took aspirin during their pregnancy, and 1,515 mother-child pairs were classified as "heavily exposed." They found no association between aspirin intake and low birth weight or perinatal mortality. These authors, and Collins and Turner in a subsequent letter to the Editor of Lancet, comment on the possible causes for the discrepancy in findings including sample size, amount of salicylate ingested, verification of salicylate use, and patient selection.

Salicylates can prolong both pregnancy and labor in rats. A similar association has been suggested in the human in retrospective analysis of aspirin users taking daily doses of 3 gm or over. In addition, an increased incidence of antepartum and postpartum hemorrhage was noted. The hemorrhagic tendencies can also be observed in the newborn of aspirin users. Abnormal platelet function and decreases in factor XII occur, possibly leading to hemorrhages in the infants. In view of its ability to compete with bilirubin for albumin binding sites, aspirin may predispose the newborn to a greater likelihood of bilirubin toxicity, especially in the presence of isoimmunization.

In conclusion, there is no firm evidence that aspirin is teratogenic in the human. If there is such an effect, it is apparently weak in view of the widespread use of this compound. The hematologic alterations, however, should be considered; and changes described in newborns are consistent with our own observations. It seems prudent, therefore, when possible, to avoid high doses and prolonged usage of salicylates during pregnancy, and to discontinue the drug when labor is anticipated. Again, no matter the dose, aspirin is best avoided, particularly during the first 10 weeks of gestation. In any case, as with all medications, its use should be confined to definite indications, utilizing the minimal effective dose.

Methadone

The pharmacokinetics of heroin and methadone are different, and results indicate decided advantages in bringing pregnant women into methadone treatment programs. Obstetric complications appear less often in pregnant addicts receiving methadone therapy than in untreated heroin addicts.

Methadone crosses the placental barrier, although the maternal plasma levels are higher than those in the cord blood or the amniotic fluid. There is no consistent relationship between the dose of methadone and the levels in the maternal plasma. In pregnant patients on daily maintenance doses of methadone (30-100 mg), recorded concentrations of the drug ranged from .14-.48 μg/ml in maternal serum, .07-.39 μg/ml in amniotic fluid, and .03-.25 μg/ml in cord plasma. In samples taken simultaneously, the average amniotic fluid-to-maternal plasma ratio was 0.73 while the cord plasma-to-maternal plasma ratio was 0.59 (Blinick et al., 1975). Methadone can be measured in the neonate's urine for at least the first three days of life, with levels 10-60 times greater than those in the cord plasma and 1.2 to 25 times higher than those in the amniotic fluid (Harper et al., 1977).

Neonatal withdrawal symptoms occur as a result of maternal methadone treatment and are generally less severe than those in the neonates of heroin addicts. There is a positive correlation between the severity (but not the time of onset) of methadone withdrawal symptoms and 1) the total amount of methadone taken during the final twelve weeks of pregnancy; 2) the maternal daily dose at the time of delivery; and 3) the intrapartum maternal serum methadone levels. The newborn is likely to exhibit moderate to severe withdrawal symptoms when the maternal daily intake of methadone is 30 mg or greater, although symptoms are also observed at lower dosages. It should be noted that the intensity of the withdrawal symptoms in the newborn can be influenced by the multiplicity of maternal drug abuse. Late withdrawal symptoms occur in babies born to methadone-treated mothers probably secondary to the slow release of methadone bound to tissues.

In the reports reviewed there is no increased incidence of congenital abnormalities with the use of methadone. Nevertheless, the lowest possible dose should be utilized. The effect of methadone on birthweight is not entirely resolved; however, it appears that the lower birthweight sometimes noted may be due to factors other than the drug itself (e.g., multiple drug abuse).

Wilson (1975) showed that at birth the length and head circumferences of 29 infants exposed to well-regulated programs were normal. This is in contrast to infants born to mothers addicted to heroin (30) or to those born to mothers with limited maintenance or unprescribed use (10). In infants of heroin-addicted mothers, the incidences of length and head circumference measurements below the tenth percentile were 14 and 25%, respectively. In mothers with limited maintenance or unprescribed use, the corresponding incidences were 20 and 30%. In his follow-up study (9-36 mos) of these infants, Wilson noted that there was a decrease in the weight, height, and head circumference of infants from both heroin-addicted and methadone-treated mothers. These findings are in contrast to those reported by Blinick et al. (1975) who found normal physical and intellectual development in 14 infants (age 4½-42 mos) of methadone-treated mothers. The numbers of subjects in both studies are small; and clearly, more data with appropriate controls are needed to resolve the issue.

Disulfiram

Disulfiram is a therapeutic adjunct in chronic alcoholism. There are scant data about its use during pregnancy. In a letter to the editor of *Lancet,* Nora and associates (1977) reported severe limb reduction abnormalities in two infants whose mothers had received disulfiram during the first trimester. Alcohol and other drugs were not taken during this time. They cite another report of five pregnancies which resulted in two infants with clubfeet, two normal infants, and one spontaneous abortion.

Pregnant rats given high dosages of disulfiram (100 mg daily) from day 3 to days 12 or 13 result in a high incidence (83%) of fetal resorption. At lower dosages, 50 mg/day from day 3 to day 21, fetal resorption did not occur and no gross malformations were reported. Similarly, no fetal resorption or gross malformation occurred in rats given 100 mg/day after the 8th day (Salgo and Oster, 1974).

In rats, a copper-deficient diet produces a high rate of fetal resorption. A mechanism by which disulfiram induces fetal resorption may relate to copper deficiency since the drug chelates with copper.

The limited data on disulfiram in pregnancy preclude a definite statement about its teratogenic potential and present the clinician with a therapeutic dilemma since alcohol itself is suspected of possessing teratogenic properties. We would recommend at this time, however, that the optimal treatment of chronic alcoholism in pregnancy should include psychological and emotional therapy, without the use of disulfiram.

References and Recommended Reading

Blatman, S: Methadone and children (Commentary) Pediatrics 48:173, 1971.

Bleyer, WA, Breckenridge, RT: Studies on the detection of adverse drug reactions in the newborn. II. The effects of prenatal aspirin on newborn hemostasis. JAMA 213:2049, 1970.

Blinick, G: Fertility of narcotics addicts and effects of addiction on the offspring. Soc Biol 18(Suppl):34S, 1971.

Blinick, G, Inturrisi, CE, Jerez, E, Wallach, RC: Amniotic fluid methadone in women maintained on methadone. Mt Sinai J Med 41:254, 1974.

Blinick, G, Inturrisi, CE, Jerez, E, Wallach, RC: Methadone assays in pregnancy women and progeny. Am J Obstet Gynecol 121:617, 1975.

Blinick, G, Jerez, E, Wallach, RC: Methadone maintenance, pregnancy, and progeny. JAMA 225:477, 1973.

Blinick, G, Wallach, RC, Jerez, E: Pregnancy in narcotics addicts treated by medical withdrawal. Am J Obstet Gynecol 105:997, 1969.

Buchan, PC, MacDonald, HN: Aspirin in pregnancy. (Letter) Lancet 2:147, 1979.

Challis, RE, Scopes, JW: Late withdrawal symptoms in babies born to methadone addicts. Lancet 2:1230, 1977. (Letter)

Collins, E, Turner, G: Aspirin during pregnancy. (Letter) Lancet 2:797, 1976.

Corby, DG: Aspirin in pregnancy: Maternal and fetal effects. Pediatrics 62:930, 1978.

Davis, MM, Shanks, B: Neurological aspects of perinatal narcotic addiction and methadone treatment. Addict Dis 2:213, 1975.

Dole, VP, Nyswander, M: A medical treatment for diacetylmorphine (heroin) addiction. JAMA 193:80, 1965.

Geber, WF, Schramm, LC: Comparative teratogenicity of morphine, heroin, and methadone in the hamster. Pharmacologist 11:248, 1969.

Harper, RG, Solish, G, Feingold, E, Gersten-Woolf, NB, Sokal, MM: Maternal ingested methadone, body fluid methadone, and the neonatal withdrawal syndrome. Am J Obstet Gynecol 129:417, 1977.

Haslam, RR: Neonatal purpura secondary to maternal salicylism. J Pediatr 86:653, 1975.

Hertz, R: Discussion: Addiction, fertility, and pregnancy. Soc Biol 18(Suppl):40S, 1971.

Heymann, MA, Rudolph, AM: Effects of acetylsalicylic acid on the ductus arteriosus and circulation in fetal lambs in utero. Circulation Res 38:418, 1976.

Inturrisi, CE, Blinick, G, Lipsitz, PJ: Methadone levels in human maternal, fetal, and newborn biofluids. Pharmacologist 15:168, 1973.

Kandall, SR, Gartner, LM: Late presentation of drug withdrawal symptoms in newborns. Am J Dis Child 127:58, 1974.

Khera, KS: Teratogenicity studies with methotrexate, aminopterin, and acetylsalicylic acid in domestic cats. Teratology 14:21, 1976.

Kwentus, J, Major, LF: Disulfiram in the treatment of alcoholism. A review. J Stud Alcohol 40:428, 1979.

Lipsitz, PJ, Blatman, S: Newborn infants of mothers on methadone maintenance. NY State J Med 74:994, 1974.

Lubaway, WC, Garrett, RJB: Effects of aspirin and acetaminophen on fetal and placental growth in rats. J Pharm Sci 66:111, 1977.

McLaughlin, PJ, Zagon, I, White, WJ: Perinatal methadone exposure in rats. Effects on body and organ development. Biol Neonate 34:48, 1978.

McNiel, JR: The possible teratogenic effect of salicylates on the developing fetus. Clinical Pediatr 12:347, 1973.

Nora, AH, Nora, JJ, Blu, J: Limb-reduction anomalies in infants born to disulfiram-treated alcoholic mothers. Lancet 2:664, 1977.

Ostrea, EM, Chavez, CJ: Perinatal problems (excluding neonatal withdrawal) in maternal drug addiction: A study of 830 cases. J Pediatr 94:292, 1979.

Pierson, PS, Howard, P, Kleber, HD: Sudden deaths in infants born to methadone-maintained addicts. JAMA 220:1733, 1972.

Rajegowda, BK, Glass, L, Evans, HE, Maso, G, Swartz, DP, Leblanc, W: Methadone withdrawal in newborn infants. J Pediatr 81:532, 1972.

Reddy, AM, Harper, RG, Stern, G: Observations on heroin and methadone withdrawal in the newborn. Pediatrics 48:353, 1971.

Rosen, TS, Pippenger, CE: Pharmacologic observations on the neonatal withdrawal syndrome. J Pediatr 88:1044, 1976.

Salgo, MP, Oster, G: Fetal resorption induced by disulfiram in rats. J Reprod Fert 39:375, 1974.

Shapiro, S, Monson, RR, Kaufman, DW, et al.: Perinatal mortality and birthweight in relation to aspirin taken during pregnancy. Lancet 1:1375, 1976.

Slone, D, Heinonen, OP, Kaufman, DW, et al.: Aspirin and congenital malformations. Lancet 1:1373, 1976.

Strauss, ME, Andresko, M, Stryker, JC, Wardell, JN, Dunkel, LD: Methadone maintenance during pregnancy: Pregnancy, birth, and neonatal characteristics. Am J Obstet Gynecol 120:895, 1975.

Turner, G, Collins, E: Fetal effects of regular salicylate ingestion in pregnancy. Lancet 2:338, 1975.

Wallach, RC, Jerez, E, Blinick, G: Pregnancy and menstrual function in narcotics addicts treated with methadone. Am J Obstet Gynecol 105:1226, 1969.

Wilson, G: Somatic growth effects of perinatal addiction. Addict Dis 2:333, 1975.

Wilson, JG, Ritter, EJ, Scott, WJ, Fradkin, R: Comparative distribution and embryotoxicity of acetylsalicylic acid in pregnant rats and rhesus monkeys. Toxicol Appl Pharmacol 41:67, 1977.

Zelson, C, Lee, SJ, Casalino, M: Neonatal narcotic addiction. Comparative effects of maternal intake of heroin and methadone. N Eng J Med 289:1216, 1973.

PSYCHOTROPIC DRUGS

Howard J. Osofsky, M.D., Ph.D.

*Staff and Research Psychiatrist
The Menninger Foundation;
Clinical Professor of Obstetrics and Gynecology
University of Kansas Medical Center
Kansas City, Kansas*

In considering the use of psychotropic drugs during pregnancy, it is important to evaluate the various categories of psychotropic drugs separately and to be aware of the indications, contraindications and complications that can occur within each. However, in beginning this section a general statement would appear worthwhile. Despite widespread clinical experience with prescribed psychotropic medications in humans, a surprising paucity of complications directly attributable to these drugs has been observed. Although the Food and Drug Administration has now advised caution in the use of many psychotropic drugs during pregnancy, and although no careful physician would prescribe psychotropic medications for pregnant women (especially during the first trimester) unless there were well-substantiated indications for the drug, generally it would appear that the majority of these medications are relatively safe for the mother and her unborn fetus when they are properly prescribed.

Antipsychotic Drugs

Commonly referred to as neuroleptics or "major tranquilizers" these agents differ from other psychotropic drugs in both their capacity to ameliorate schizophrenic symptoms and the occurrence of extrapyramidal side effects. Four groups of antipsychotic drugs are used in the United States. These include:
A. Phenothiazines, B. Butyrophenones, C. Thioxanthenes, D. Oxoindoles

Phenothiazines are most commonly classified into:
1. Aliphatics, including chlorpromazine, promazine, triflupromazine.
2. Piperazines, including acetophenazine, fluphenazine, perphenazine, prochlorperazine, carphenazine, trifluoperazine, thiopropazate and butaperazine.
3. Piperidines, including thioridazine, piperacetazine and mesoridazine.

It is noteworthy that one of the piperazines, prochlorperazine, was widely prescribed until recently as an antiemetic during early pregnancy. Some of the differences among the three groups of phenothiazines are: The *aliphatics* are accompanied by relatively more sedation, hypotension, dermatitis and convulsions but less extrapyramidal side effects. The *piperazines* are accompanied by more extrapyramidal side effects but less sedation, hypotension and lens opacities. The *piperidines* are accompanied by the lowest incidences of extrapyramidal side effects, but higher incidences of retinal toxicity, ejaculatory disturbances and electrocardiography effects. Phenothiazines help bring hypo- and hyperactivity to more normal levels, assist with patient socialization and over a period of several weeks, aid in the elimination of thought disorder. Side effects of treatment include initial drowsiness which is common but of relatively short duration, akathisia (or motor restlessness), acute dystonias, drowsiness, dry mouth, weight gain, postural hypotension, skin rash, phototoxicity, jaundice and hyperhydrosis.

The significance of some of these symptoms during pregnancy should be emphasized. Although akathisia and acute dystonias are clinically problematic, it is worth noting that if patients use lozenges for dry mouth, they should be sugarless because superimposed monilia infections are common. Problems with weight gain may be particularly burdensome during pregnancy, since the weight gain can be hard to treat and can be resistant to general dietary measures. Although chlorpromazine may interfere with bilirubin metabolism by binding serum albumin, evidence of accentuated neonatal jaundice or liver toxicity due to chlorpromazine during pregnancy is not documented in the literature. Although reports have been published concerning possible teratogenic effects of phenothiazines, there is no well-documented evidence of increased incidences of either chromosomal abnormalities or fetal damage following the use of these drugs during human pregnancy. Extrapyramidal symptoms have occasionally been reported in newborns following maternal use of phenothiazines (Ananth, 1976; Ayd, 1968; Cleary, 1977; Hill, 1966; Tamer et al., 1969). Although relatively uncommon, these symptoms may persist until six months of age. Infants should be observed and treated if these symptoms develop.

Butyrophenones are most commonly represented in this country by haloperidol but include trifluperidol and droperidol, which is more commonly used in anesthesia. Haloperidol is claimed to be helpful in patients with paranoid ideation, agitation and withdrawal. Extrapyramidal side effects are quite common, but autonomic effects and allergic reactions are rare.

Thioxanthenes are represented by chlorprothixene and thiothixene. Clinical effectiveness is similar to the phenothiazines.

Oxoindoles represented by molindone, are also therapeutically similar to the phenothiazines. Occasional cases of severe limb malformations have been reported following maternal use of haloperidol early in the first trimester of pregnancy (Kopelman et al., 1975). It has been suggested that days 25-37 may be of special importance because of the timing of the limb development in humans, and that the specificity in timing of the insult may explain the relative paucity of reporting cases of deformity. It should be emphasized that reports remain sporadic at present, and documentation of a link between maternal ingestion of haloperidol and fetal limb deformities has not been well-established.

A number of other findings would appear worthy of note. The antipsychotic drugs may be accompanied by false increases in determinations of alkaline phosphates, urine and serum bilirubin, porphyrins, transaminase and urobilinogen. Fasting glucose levels may possibly be falsely elevated. Urinary estrogen assessments may be inaccurate, as may 17-hydroxysteroid and protein-bound iodine determinations.

Various phenothiazine preparations are excreted in breast milk. Chlorpromazine, thioridazine, mesoridazine, prochlorperazine and trifluoperazine are transmitted in relatively small amounts. It has been reported that a daily dose of chlorpromazine must be 200 mg. or more for the drug to enter breast milk, and that even with high doses the presence of chlorpromazine in breast milk is barely detectable (Uhlif and Ryznar, 1973; Blacker et al., 1962). It appears probable that the quantities of phenothiazines excreted in breast milk are harmless to the neonate (Ananth, 1978). We might note that haloperidol is excreted in slightly greater amounts in breast milk. Although animal studies have suggested that neonates may develop behavioral symptoms when their mothers are taking haloperidols, human clinical documentation of side effects in the breast-fed neonates of mothers receiving this drug has not been established.

Drugs Used to Treat Depression

These include the tricyclic derivatives and the MAO inhibitors. The commonly used tricyclic derivatives are: imipramine, desipramine, amitriptyline, nortriptyline, protriptyline and doxepin. The MAO inhibitors commonly used include: hydrazides, including isocarboxazid and phenalzine, and the non-hydrazides, represented by tranylcypromine. These drugs are primarily used for the depressive syndromes. These include unipolar depressive disorders, encompassing endogenous or autonomous depression, chronic characterological depression, agitated "involutional" depression, and situational (reactive) depressions, manic-depressive (bipolar) disorders, and in some situations schizoid-affective disorders. In the case of manic depressive (bipolar) disorders, lithium carbonate may also be very useful clinically. Symptoms usually improve within one month following administration of the drugs. In general, "endogenous" depressions appear to respond better to tricyclic antidepressants than do "reactive" depressions. If the drugs are not effective using adequate doses after one month of treatment, consideration should be given to the use of MAO inhibitors or, occasionally, electroconvulsive therapy. MAO inhibitors are sometimes superior to the tricyclic antidepressants in phobic anxiety states. Side effects of tricyclic antidepressants include minor central nervous system symptoms such as agitation, fine tremor, anger, drowsiness, awkwardness and sudden falls, autonomic nervous system effects (primarily of an anticholinergic nature) and cardiovascular effects with occasional flattened T-waves on EKGs. If patients are taking MAO inhibitors, they need to be cautioned about serious side effects including dangerous synergism with other drugs. Hypertensive crises may occur if patients eat foods with tyramine such as cheese, wine (especially sherry and chianti), beer, pickled herring, yeast extracts, chicken liver, cream, chocolate and fava beans. The first symptom may be unusual and severe headaches.

While patients are taking antidepressants, especially tricyclics, the alkaline phosphatase, bilirubin, and transaminase levels may be falsely elevated; BSP retention may be increased; and fasting blood sugar levels may either be falsely increased or decreased.

Considering the huge amount of antidepressants that have been prescribed, there is surprisingly little information available concerning potential adverse effects in human pregnancy. There is no firm evidence to substantiate increased incidences of either chromosomal abnormalities or spontaneous abortions. Occasional reports exist associating tricyclic antidepressants with limb-reduction deformities and other malformations. However, data from more extensive national surveys do not substantiate the tricyclics as a cause of such abnormalities (DiMascio and Goldberg, 1976). In general, most studies have recorded little or no tricyclic excretion in breask milk. Therefore, it appears that nursing is not contraindicated in women taking tricyclic antidepressants. There have been occasional reports of infants whose mothers had been taking the drug during pregnancy having withdrawal symptoms during the first thirty days of life (Ananth, 1976; Webster, 1973). These symptoms included dyspnea, cyanosis, tachypnea, tachycardia, irritability and profuse sweating. The physician should be aware of the possibility of such symptoms occurring, although according to the reports they disappeared spontaneously without apparent sequelae.

Lithium carbonate has been a particularly useful adjunct in the treatment of manic-depressive (bipolar) disorders. More recently it has been suggested that the drug can be useful as an adjunct in treating patients with diagnoses of borderline personality organization and schizophrenia, especially when there is an affective component in the patients' emotional difficulty. Some have suggested its usefulness as an adjunct in the treatment of postpartum depression. When patients are first placed on the drug, they commonly experience mild gastrointestinal disturbances; they may feel tired or sleepy and experience muscular weakness; they may note hand tremor, and they may be aware of thirst and need for frequent urination. These symptoms are usually mild and generally subside in several days. More persistent side reactions which may develop over time include hand tremor, polydipsia and polyuria, weight gain and non-toxic goiter. When goiter occurs, it is usually mild and can be reduced by thyroxin; however, it is important to watch for the exacerbation of latent hypothyroidism. Long-term renal damage may occur, so renal function should be monitored in patients receiving lithium for an extended period of time. The maintenance dosage of lithium should be the lowest that produces clinical results.

The use of lithium during pregnancy remains open to question. Some reviewers have concluded that there is no increased incidence of congenital malformations in babies born to lithium-treated mothers (DiMascio and Goldberg, 1976). However, a number of reports have suggested the possibility of increased incidences of fetal abnormalities, especially cardiovascular abnormalities (Weinstein and Goldfield, 1975). Ebstein's anomaly, with distortion and displacement of the tricuspid valve and secondary abnormalities of the right ventricle and atrium and possible atrial septal defects or patent foramen ovale, has been described in a number of infants whose mothers received the drug. Therefore, although the majority of data suggests that lithium carbonate is safe during pregnancy, it would seem prudent to avoid using the drug during pregnancy where possible, especially during the first trimester. Since childbirth may precipitate the reappearance of mania, it has been suggested that lithium carbonate—if discontinued—be resumed during the last trimester of pregnancy (Targum et al., 1979).

When lithium carbonate is employed during pregnancy, careful attention must be given to regulation of dosage. Lithium clearance by the renal system tends to increase as pregnancy advances. Therefore, the patient may have decreases in serum lithium concentrations with previously satisfactory doses. It has been advised that the dose of lithium be decreased by 50% during the last week of pregnancy, discontinued at the onset of labor, and then reinstated at prepregnancy doses in the immediate postpartum period. Since sodium loss tends to be associated with increased lithium concentration, patients receiving lithium should not be placed on sodium-restricted diets or given diuretics during pregnancy.

There have been occasional reports of lithium toxicity in newborns whose mothers had been receiving the drug (Ananth, 1976; Burgess, 1979; Tunnessen and Hertz, 1972). The toxic effects have included unusual flaccidity, cyanosis and a transient heart murmur. One infant has been described with generalized edema and a large goiter born to a mother with a slight goiter before lithium treatment, but whose goiter grew much larger during the course of treatment in pregnancy. The infant's edema disappeared in a few days and the goiter disappeared almost completely within two months. Lithium is excreted in breast milk in concentrations of ¼ to ½ of maternal serum levels. For this reason, it would appear advisable to discourage breast feeding in mothers receiving lithium treatment (Ananth, 1978).

Anti-Anxiety Drugs

The anti-anxiety drugs (minor tranquilizers) are among the most widely prescribed drugs by physicians. They are commonly used for anxiety reactions where they appear to be effective, but are often not needed. They may also be of use in a number of other reactive situations, for example, for anxiety accompanying phobias around such conditions as separation and travel. Three common groups of anti-anxiety drugs are employed:

A. Glycerol derivatives, B. Benzodiazepines, C. Diphenylmethane derivatives.

The common glycerol derivatives are meprobamate and tybamate. The common benzodiazepines in use are chlordiazepoxide, diazepam, oxazepam, clorazepate dipotassium and flurazepam hydrochloride. The diphenylmethane derivative in common use is hydroxyzine. The anti-anxiety drugs tend to reduce manifest anxiety and somatic complaints. They also have sedative, anticonvulsant and muscle relaxant properties. They do not ameliorate schizophrenic symptoms and do not produce extrapyramidal side effects. Their effects are potentiated by alcohol and central nervous system depressants; patients should be warned about drinking or combining anti-anxiety and sedative drugs. The benzodiazepines have been very effective in suppressing symptoms of alcohol withdrawal. The diphenylmethane derivative, hydroxyzine, has been used relatively widely to provide sedation and a decrease in anxiety during labor.

In general, the anti-anxiety drugs seem relatively safe for use in pregnancy. First trimester use of diazepam has been linked in two studies to a higher incidence of cleft lip and possibly of cleft palate (Safra and Oakley, 1975; Saxen and Saxen, 1975). However, other reports have not substantiated this increased risk. Similarly, meprobamate-containing drugs and chlordiazepoxide have been associated with increased incidences of spontaneous abortions and fetal anomalies (Milkovich and Van Den Berg, 1974). However, a large-scale follow-up study was unable to substantiate any such abnormalities or long-term difficulties in infants whose mothers received these drugs during pregnancy (Hartz et al., 1975). Thus although prudence is warranted in prescribing anti-anxiety drugs during pregnancy, especially during the first trimester, current evidence does not definitively link the use of these drugs with the development of fetal abnormalities.

Cases have been reported of withdrawal symptoms in newborn infants whose mothers took considerable quantities of anti-anxiety medication during pregnancy (Lawson and Wilson, 1979; Patrick et al., 1972; Prenner, 1977; Rementeria and Bhatt, 1977). The symptoms have been similar to those reported with narcotic withdrawal: jitteriness, tachypnea, poor suck and feeding, irritability, clonic movements and shrill cry. Persistence of these symptoms may occur for some weeks following delivery. Chlordiazepoxide is excreted in breast milk in modest quantities. Although these quantities are not usually considered sufficient to affect infants, central depression may occur. Diazepam is also excreted in breast milk in small quantities. However, in one study the levels of diazepam and its metabolites in neonatal blood decreased after four days, suggesting diminished neonatal susceptibility after that time (Erkkola and Kanto, 1972). It has also been emphasized that the detoxification of diazepam is accomplished by its conjugation with glucuronic acid, the same mechanism by which free bilirubin is eliminated. It is possible that if infants receive diazepam through breast milk or from other sources, physiological jaundice may be prolonged and hyperbilirubinemia may occur (Ananth, 1978). As a result, some have suggested that it is inadvisable to give diazepam to nursing mothers. Chlorazepate may cause drowsiness in infants of nursing mothers; it is therefore suggested that this drug not be administered during nursing. Meprobamate is excreted in appreciable amounts in breast milk and the concentration of this drug in breast milk can vary between half and four times that in maternal plasma. Although meprobamate is usually a relatively safe, non-toxic drug, infants or nursing mothers who are receiving this drug should be monitored for possible signs of drug intoxication.

References and Recommended Reading

Ananth, J: Side effects on fetus and infant of psychotropic drug use during pregnancy. Int Pharmacopsychiat 11:246, 1976.

Ananth, J: Side effects in the neonate from psychotropic agents excreted through breast-feeding. Am J Psychiat 135:801, 1978.

Ayd, FJ: Phenothiazine therapy during pregnancy. Int Ther Newsl 3:39, 1968.

Blacker, KH, Weinstein, BJ, Ellman, GL: Mothers' milk and chlorpromazine. Am J Psychiat 119:178, 1962.

Burgess, HA: When a patient on lithium is pregnant. Am J Nurs 1989, 1979.

Cleary, MF: Fluphenazine decanoate during pregnancy. Am J Psychiat. 134:815, 1977.

Cooper, SJ: Psychotropic drugs in pregnancy: morphological and psychological adverse effects on offspring. J Biosoc Sci 10:321, 1978.

Crombie, DL, Pinsent, RJ, Fleming, DM et al.: Fetal effects of tranquilizers in pregnancy. N Engl J Med 293:198, 1975.

DiMascio, A and Goldberg, HL: Emotional disorders: An outline guide to diagnosis and pharmacological treatment. Oradell, New Jersey, Medical Economics, 1976.

Erkkola, R, Kanto, J: Diazepam and breast-feeding. Lancet 1:1235, 1972.

Goldberg, HL and DiMascio, A: Psychotropic drugs in pregnancy. In Psychopharmacology: A generation of progress. M.A. Lipton, A. Dimascio and K.F. Killam (Eds.) New York, Raven Press, 1978, p. 1047.

Hartz, SC, Heinonen, OP, Shapiro, S, Siskind, V and Slone, D: Antenatal exposure to meprobamate and chlordiazepoxide in relation to malformations, mental development, and childhood mortality. N Engl J Med 292:726, 1975.

Hill, RM, Desmond, MM, and Kay, JL: Extrapyramidal dysfunction in an infant of a schizophrenic mother. J Pediat 69:589, 1966.

Kopelman, AE, McCullar, FW, Heggeness, L: Limb malformations following maternal use of haloperidol. JAMA 231:62, 1975.

Lawson, MS and Wilson, GS: Addiction and pregnancy: Two lives in crisis. Social Work in Health Care 4:445, 1979.

Milkovich, L and Van Den Berg, BJ: Effects of prenatal meprobamate and chlordiazepoxide hydrochloride on human embryonic and fetal development. N Engl J Med 291:1268, 1974.

Patrick, NJ, Tilstone, WJ, Reavey, P: Diazepam and breast-feeding. Lancet 1:542, 1972.

Prenner, Bruce M: Neonatal withdrawal syndrome associated with hydroxyzine hydrochloride. Am J Dis Child 131:529, 1977.

Rementeria, JL and Bhatt, K: Withdrawal symptoms in neonates from intrauterine exposure to diazepam. J Pediat 90:123, 1977.

Safra, MJ and Oakley, GP: Association between cleft lip with or without cleft palate and prenatal exposure to diazepam. Lancet 2:478, 1975.

Saxen, I, Saxen, L: Letter: Association between maternal intake of diazepam and oral clefts. Lancet 2:498, 1975.

Silbermann, RM, Beenen, F and de Jong, H: Clinical treatment of postpartum delirium with perfenazine and lithium carbonate. Psychiatria Clin 8:314, 1975.

Tamer, A, McKey, R, Arias, D, Worly, L and Fogel, BJ: Phenothiazine-induced extrapyramidal dysfunction in the neonate. J Pediat 75:479, 1969.

Targum, SD, Davenport, YB and Webster, MJ: Brief communication: Postpartum mania in bipolar manic-depressive patients withdrawn from lithium carbonate. J Nerv Ment Dis 167:572, 1979.

Tunnessen, WW and Hertz, CG: Toxic effects of lithium in newborn infants: A commentary. J Pediat 81:804, 1972.

Uhlif, F and Ryznar, J: Appearance of chlorpromazine in mothers' milk. Activitas Nervosa Superior 15:106, 1973.

Webster, PAC: Withdrawal symptoms in neonates associated with maternal antidepressant therapy. Lancet 2:318, 1973.

Weinstein, MR and Goldfield, MD: Cardiovascular malformations with lithium use during pregnancy. Am J Psychiat 132:5, 1975.

4

EFFECTS OF BIOLOGICALLY FOREIGN COMPOUNDS ON REPRODUCTION

DONALD R. MATTISON, M.D.

Pregnancy Research Branch
National Institute of Child Health and Human Development
National Institutes of Health
Bethesda, MD 20205

Reproduction begins with gametogenesis in the male and female, continues with gamete interaction or fertilization, and is completed with the development and sexual maturation of the newly formed individual (Fig. 1). These reproductive processes do not take place in a chemically pristine environment, but rather in an environment which is increasingly contaminated with the products and by-products of the chemical age in which we live. Certain environmental pollutants are known to be toxic, carcinogenic, or mutagenic. A smaller number of xenobiotic compounds have been demonstrated to impair reproduction in experimental animals or humans. The vast majority of xenobiotics, however, have not been carefully tested for toxicity to the reproductive system.

Reproduction is a complex process requiring many levels of control. Figure 1 lists only some of the steps in the reproductive process, and does not indicate control mechanisms. The biology of toxicology is similarly complex; it involves absorption, distribution, metabolism (toxification and/or detoxification), excretion and repair.

The issue of species differentiation in both reproduction and

REPRODUCTIVE CYCLE

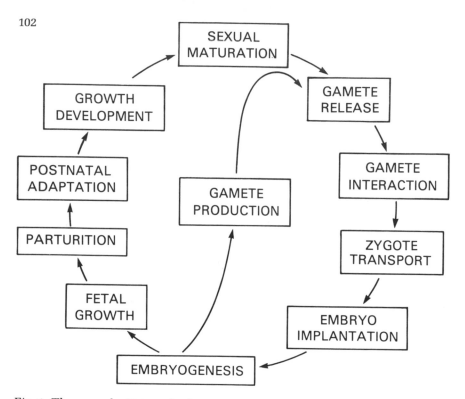

Fig. 1. The reproductive cycle, from gametogenesis to sexual maturation. This cycle illustrates the complex multi-stage process of reproduction in mammalian species.

toxicology is dependent on mechanisms of hormonal control, anatomy, pharmacokinetics, metabolism, etc. In some instances these species differences are poorly understood. A reproductive toxin in one species may not be toxic in another (including humans) because of differences in reproductive or toxicologic mechanisms. Some of the toxins discussed in this chapter are known to affect human reproduction, others are presented as examples of additional mechanisms of toxicity, without knowledge of human susceptibility. The teratogenicity of thalidomide is an instructive example of species susceptibility, in that rat and mouse are insensitive, while rabbit, human and non-human primates are sensitive (Shepard, 1976).

Another pertinent issue in toxicology concerns possible gender differences in toxicity (Doull, 1975). This is also crucial in reproductive toxicology because of differences in biological mechanisms of reproduction in males and females. As a result of the accessibility of gametes and gonads, more compounds have been demonstrated to be toxic in males than in females. At the present time it is not known if this represents an actual gender difference in gonadal or gamete toxicity.

Because reproduction is essential for continued existence of any species, it is clearly necessary to develop an understanding of reproductive toxins: mechanisms of action, site of action, as well as species (especially human) susceptibility. Impaired reproductive capability among patients may result from occupational or environmental exposures (dibromochloropropane, halogenated hydrocarbons), personal habits (smoking or alcohol abuse), or drug treatment (cimetidine, cyclophosphamide). General aspects of testicular (Lucier et al., 1977) and ovarian toxicity (Mattison, 1980) have been addressed, and a recent conference was devoted to gonadal toxicity (Dixon, 1978).

Unfortunately, many human reproductive toxins have been identified by the exposed individuals rather than by health professionals (see discussion of dibromochloropropane). This suggests the need for careful research stimulated by *the most essential element of human biology, an inquisitive physician, alert to the diverse etiologies of disease.*

MECHANISMS OF TOXICITY

The mechanisms of toxicity can be reduced ultimately to an effect which interrupts the normal functioning of a cell, organ or organism (Casarett and Doull, 1975). This toxic effect may be very specific, affecting only a single function of a single cell type, or broad and nonspecific with multiple sites of toxicity within an organism.

Reproductive toxins may act directly (Fig. 2) either by virtue of structural similarity to an endogenous compound (i.e., hormone, nutrient), or because of chemical reactivity (i.e., alkylating agent, denaturant, chelator). Or they may act indirectly, requiring metabolic activation within the organism or organ before exerting a toxic effect. The metabolite formed may then exert its toxic effect through one of the direct mechanisms of reproductive toxicity described (structural similarity or chemical reactivity). Other indirect acting reproductive toxins may produce alterations in physiological control mechanisms of the organism (i.e., enzyme induction or inhibition).

Direct Acting Toxins

Structural Similarity: One mechanism of direct acting reproductive toxins results from structural similarity to a biologically

MECHANISMS OF REPRODUCTIVE TOXICITY

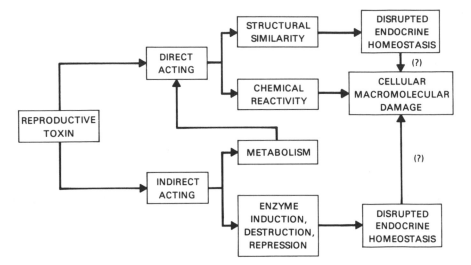

Fig. 2. Mechanisms of reproductive toxicity. Each of the mechanisms suggested above is represented by one or more of the toxins discussed in the text.

active molecule. These compounds may best be considered wolves in sheeps' clothing, in that they can mislead an organism. The compounds in this category are generally agonists or antagonists of endogenous hormones. A well-known example of this type of direct acting "reproductive toxin" are the oral contraceptives which act predominantly by suppression of gonadotropin secretion. Occupational exposure to oral contraceptives, for example during formulation, represents an obvious example of a reproductive and endocrine toxin (Harrington et al., 1978). The direct acting reproductive toxins considered here are cimetidine and diethylstilbestrol.

Chemical Reactivity: Compounds which are chemically reactive are usually nonspecific in their site of action. Because of chemical reactivity, exposure to these compounds generally results from occupational exposure or drug treatment. The examples considered here are alkylating agents found in the chemical industry and used in the treatment of many neoplastic and some non-neoplastic human diseases. Because of their reactivity most of these compounds are toxic, carcinogenic, or mutagenic in other organ systems, and their reproductive toxicity has often been overlooked. Other examples of direct acting reproductive toxins presented are cadmium and boron.

Indirect Acting Toxins

Metabolic Activation: In addition to direct interference with reproductive processes, certain toxins may act indirectly to impair reproduction, for example, those toxins which are metabolized to form a toxic metabolite. The metabolites formed may be chemically reactive or may mimic an endogenous molecule.

One of the mechanisms utilized to remove hydrophobic xenobiotics from the body is oxidation by microsomal monooxygenases; this increases the polarity of the molecule. The polar metabolite is then conjugated or excreted directly. Unfortunately, some of the metabolites formed in this process are chemically reactive. These reactive metabolites formed *in vivo* may then interact with cellular macromolecules just as exogenously administered chemically reactive compounds. This mechanism results in the reproductive toxicity of cyclophosphamide, dibromochloropropane, and the polycyclic aromatic hydrocarbons.

The ovary and testis have been demonstrated to have the microsomal monooxygenases responsible for metabolic activation of many xenobiotic compounds (Mattison and Thorgeirsson, 1978, 1979; Dixon and Lee, 1980).

Enzyme Modification: Other indirect acting reproductive toxins may induce or inhibit enzyme systems important in reproduction—enhancing or suppressing steroid secretion or clearance. Because reproduction requires hormonal feedback loops for successful control, xenobiotics which alter the rate of steroid synthesis or clearance may alter reproductive processes. This has been demonstrated in rodents treated with several of the halogenated polycyclic hydrocarbon pesticides discussed in this chapter, including DDT, polychlorinated biphenyls and polybrominated biphenyls.

Detoxification

Biological organisms have several mechanisms available for responding to toxic stresses. These mechanisms are classified as detoxification mechanisms and exhibit a relatively broad specificity as would be expected from the wide range of chemicals dealt with (Aitio, 1978; Oesch, 1972).

Detoxification mechanisms represent an immediate cellular response to a toxic insult and may involve conjugation with sulfate, glucuronate, or glutathione, or hydrolysis by epoxide hydratase, all acting to decrease the concentration of chemically reactive toxins within the cell. Other mechanisms of detoxification may involve metabolism of the toxin to a less toxic or more easily excreted (i.e., more polar) compound.

The mechanisms used by the cell for detoxification depend in part on the nature of the toxic molecule. Compounds that are chemically reactive, such as alkylating agents, or epoxides are detoxified by epoxide hydratase and/or conjugation systems, while non-polar compounds are first metabolized by monooxygenases to more polar products before conjugation and excretion. Some of the detoxification pathways have been demonstrated in the ovary and testis (Mukhtar et al., 1978; Lee and Dixon, 1978).

Repair

Although the cell has mechanisms for detoxification, in some instances those mechanisms provide inadequate protection resulting in cell or organ damage. When a cell or organ has been damaged by a toxin it must attempt to repair that damage.

The mechanisms of repair may be as simple as renewed or increased protein synthesis to replace nonfunctioning proteins destroyed by the toxin. More sophisticated (biologically) repair mechanisms appear to have evolved for DNA damage (Lehmann and Bridges, 1977). These mechanisms involve screening for damage in DNA, as well as several enzymes for excision of the damaged DNA region and subsequent replacement of the region excised.

Recent investigations have suggested that the mature oocyte can repair damage in oocyte DNA before and after fertilization (Pedersen and Manigia, 1978), and in sperm DNA after fertilization (Generoso et al., 1979). However, it is not known if other types of repair mechanisms exist in the oocyte. Studies by Dixon and Lee (1980) have also demonstrated DNA repair capability in the developing sperm.

REPRODUCTIVE TOXINS

Cimetidine

A good example of a direct acting reproductive toxin is the histamine (H2 receptor) antagonist, cimetidine, a drug effective in the treatment of peptic ulcer disease. An early reported side effect of cimetidine in the male was gynecomastia (Hall, 1976). Subsequent investigation in the rat demonstrated that cimetidine is an androgen antagonist, blocking the effect of exogenous androgen on seminal vesicle and prostatic weight (Winters et al., 1979).

A prospective study of men treated with cimetidine demonstrated a 43% mean reduction in sperm count after six weeks of therapy (Van Thiel et al., 1979b). These men also had increased serum testosterone and blunted response to GnRH. It is not known if the decrease in sperm count altered fertility in these men. In addition, it has been suggested that cimetidine can produce impotence in men (Wolf, 1979).

The mechanism of action of cimetidine would appear to result from competition with dihydrotestosterone for the androgen receptor (Winters et al., 1979). Since cimetidine is apparently a pure antagonist with no androgen-like (agonist) activity, the net effect is to decrease end organ responsiveness to androgen stimulation, which is consistent with the observed gynecomastia and decreased sperm counts. Cimetidine also stimulates prolactin secretion (Eversmann et al., 1979). At present, it is not known if cimetidine is able to pass the blood-testis barrier and bind to the androgen-binding protein within the seminiferous tubule or if it acts exclusively on external aspects of spermatogenesis.

Cimetidine would be a reproductive toxin in any species with a testosterone (or dihydrotestosterone) receptor similar to that in the human or rodent male. Detoxification occurs primarily by clearance and physiological readjustment.

Diethylstilbestrol

Another reproductive toxin with two possible mechanisms of action is the estrogen agonist diethylstilbestrol (DES), originally suggested as prophylaxis for complications of pregnancy (Smith, 1948). Subsequent clinical studies failed to demonstrate any therapeutic value in DES use (Dieckmann et al., 1953). Recent studies have demonstrated that DES treatment during pregnancy alters reproductive tract development in both the male and female rodent (McLachlan et al., 1975; Forsberg, 1969, 1970, 1972; Vorherr et al., 1979; Boylan, 1978) and human (Bibbo et al., 1975, 1977; Kaufman et al., 1977; Haney et al., 1979). In addition, the drug increases the risk of developing vaginal adenocarcinoma (Herbst et al., 1971).

DES illustrates well the difficulty in identifying a reproductive toxin. Although there is disagreement concerning the actual reproductive toxicity of DES, if usage of the drug were not associated with vaginal adenocarcinoma, it is doubtful whether the association with reproductive tract abnormalities would have emerged. Human male offspring exposed to DES in utero are more likely to have testicular and/or epididymal abnormalities as well as abnormal sperm and semen than are non-treated controls. It is not known if the genital and sperm abnormalities will produce subfertility in the DES-exposed men.

Female offspring exposed to DES in utero may have vaginal abnormalities. These women also appear to have irregular menses and dysmenorrhea more frequently than controls, and may be less fertile (Schmidt et al., 1980, Barnes et al., 1980; Herbst et al., 1980). Female DES offpsring may also have abnormal development of the uterus, with a small hypoplastic "T"-shaped endometrial cavity (Kaufmann et al., 1977; Haney et al., 1979). These studies suggest two possible mechanisms of DES action.

The genital tract abnormalities observed may represent a direct estrogen agonist effect resulting from the interaction of DES with estrogen receptors in the developing urogenital region which inhibits the re-epithelization of the vagina (Forsberg, 1969, 1970, 1972). It is not known if this mechanism would act through epithelial or stromal (Cuhna, 1976) estrogen receptors.

This estrogen agonist activity may also explain the disordered hypothalamic-pituitary-gonadal axis seen in these individuals. Perinatal or prenatal estrogen exposure has been demonstrated to alter hypothalamic patterning in rodents (Gorski, 1971). However, it is not known if similar effects can occur in humans. Disordered hypothalamic control will be discussed again in connection with the halogenated polycyclic hydrocarbons which also have estrogen agonist activity.

An alternative mechanism, more consistent with the observed carcinogenicity of DES, suggests that the parent compound is metabolized to a reactive intermediate. The reactive intermediate formed would then bind covalently to cellular macromolecules in the developing urogenital and hypothalamic regions, producing the observed toxicity and carcinogenicity. Similar mechanisms have been proposed for chemical carcinogens (Heidelberger, 1975; Sims and Grover, 1974). Recently DES has been demonstrated to be metabolized to a reactive intermediate capable of covalent binding to DNA (Blackburn et al., 1976), and to produce sister chromatid exchange in cultured human cells (Rudiger et al., 1979). A comprehensive series of experiments is continuing to characterize the metabolism (Metzler, 1976; Metzler and McLachlan, 1978) and estrogen agonist activity of DES (Korach et al., 1979).

These observations, while incomplete, suggest that prenatal exposure to estrogen agonists during critical developmental periods may alter the reproductive competence of adult males or females through anatomical or hormonal changes. Adult exposure to estrogen agonists will impair reproduction by altering gonadotropin release.

Alcohol

Male chronic alcoholics may have testicular atrophy (Lloyd and Williams, 1948; Van Thiel et al., 1979a), although it is not known if the effect is direct on the testis, or indirect through hypothalamic-pituitary effects. Recent experiments suggest that alcohol is a direct testicular toxin (Van Thiel et al., 1979a; Anderson et al., 1980). Hypothalamic toxicity has also been postulated to explain the impaired gonadotropin response in alcoholic males and alcohol-treated rodents. Fetal toxicity has also been demonstrated in the offspring of chronic alcoholic women (Hinckers, 1978; Ouellette et al., 1977; Jones and Smith, 1975).

Chlorcyclizine

Chlorcyclizine, a synthetic antihistamine produces testicular atrophy in rats in a dose-dependent manner (Wong and Hruban, 1972). The mechanism is thought to require metabolism to a reactive intermediate.

Azathioprine and 6-Mercaptopurine

6-Mercaptopurine, the active metabolite of azathioprine, a widely used immunosuppressive drug, has recently been demonstrated to reduce the fertility of the female offspring of rodents treated during pregnancy. The drug appears to act by producing a premature ovarian failure (Reimers et al., 1978, 1980). It is not known if the drug acts by inhibiting oogenesis, or destroys oocytes. At the present time human (male or female) gonadal susceptibility to the drug is not known. Azathioprine is known to be teratogenic and embryotoxic (Githens et al., 1965; Gross et al., 1977).

Salicylazosulfapyridine

Several reports have demonstrated reversible oligospermia, decreased sperm motility, and increased frequency of abnormal forms of sperm in men treated with salicylazosulfapyridine, a drug useful in ulcerative colitis (Levi et al., 1979; Traub et al., 1979; Toth, 1979a,b). At present the mechanism of action is uncertain, although Toth has suggested that toxicity may result from inhibition of prostaglandin synthetase.

Halogenated Polycyclic Hydrocarbons

This class of xenobiotics represents a large number of compounds which are currently used in several industrial or agricultural applications. Polychlorinated polycyclic hydrocarbons are used predominantly as pesticides and fungicides and include such compounds as DDT, aldrin, 2,4,5-T (the defoliant in Agent Orange), polychlorinated biphenyls (PCB), 2,4-D, heptachlor, chlordane and hexachlorophene. The polybrominated biphenyls (PBB) and PCB have also been used as insulators in transformers, and as flame retardants for wood. These compounds are notable for their persistence in the environment, and for their high fat solubility which results in their concentration in the higher members (i.e., domestic animals and humans) of the food chain (Kimbrough, 1974; Kupfer, 1975).

The halogenated polycyclics have been demonstrated in human and rodent tissues, maternal and fetal blood samples, placenta and breast milk (Woolley and Talens, 1971; O'Leary et al., 1970; Polishuk et al., 1970; Akiyama et al., 1975). The major source of human exposure to halogenated polycyclics results from the ingestion of contaminated food. The halogenated polycyclic hydrocarbons have been implicated as hepatotoxins, neurotoxins, carcinogens and reproductive toxins on the basis of several mechanisms of action (Kimbrough, 1974; Kupfer, 1975) including hormone agonist activity, induction of microsomal monooxygenases which alters hormone production or clearance, or metabolism to chemically reactive intermediates.

DDT (1,1,1-trichloro-2,2-bis(p-chlorophenyl)ethane), is a polychlorinated hydrocarbon which was widely used as a pesticide in the United States until it was withdrawn from the market in the early 1970's. The compound can interfere with mammalian reproduction in two ways, and may be considered a prototype for the halogenated polycyclics.

Neonatal treatment of rats with DDT produces premature vaginal opening, and subsequently results in an anovulatory syndrome similar to human polycystic ovary disease (Heinrichs et al., 1971; Gellert et al., 1972, 1974; Gellert and Heinrichs, 1975). The development of persistent estrus, as well as premature vaginal opening is dose-dependent. Rats treated with DDT also had inhibition of the normal gonadotropin elevation following ovariectomy, in a DDT dose-dependent fashion.

The mechanism of action of DDT in advancing the age of vaginal opening, producing persistent estrus, and inhibiting the rise of gonadotropins following castration is thought to result from the estrogen agonist activity of DDT (Welch et al., 1969; Bitman and Cecil, 1970). The site of action is believed to be the vagina and hypothalamus, with neonatal treatment altering the patterning of the hypothalamus (Gorski, 1971).

Similar experiments with the polychlorinated biphenyls have also demonstrated a direct relationship between the estrogen agonist activity of a molecule and its ability to advance the age of vaginal opening, and produce persistent estrus (Gellert, 1978).

These observations, together with those demonstrating transfer of the halogenated polycyclics across the placenta and through breast milk, have led to the hypothesis that human polycystic ovary disease may result from fetal and/or neonatal exposure to compounds like DDT which alter hypothalamic patterning. This hypothesis has been tested by comparing the season of birth of women with ovulatory dysfunction with that of the population as a whole (Bourne, 1974). This design was chosen because DDT usage was seasonal, beginning in late spring, peaking in summer and tapering into the fall.

Although the data for white women born in the western United States supported the hypothesis, another group of women heterogenous for race and birthplace failed to support the hypothesis. Since the mechanisms of control along the hypothalamic-pituitary-ovarian axis are different in rodents and humans, it is not surprising that the results are not conclusive. The evidence suggests, however, that prenatal or perinatal exposure to halogenated polycyclics with estrogen agonist activity may alter the hypothalamus in humans.

The halogenated hydrocarbons may also impair reproduction by another mechanism, which involves induction of hepatic and non-hepatic microsomal monooxygenases. These microsomal cytochrome P-450-dependent monooxygenases can oxygenate a wide variety of endogenous (steroids, prostaglandins, fatty acids) and exogenous (xenobiotics, drugs, pesticides) substrates (Fleischer and Packer, 1978). As previously mentioned, the role of these enzymes is to form hydrophilic products from non-polar substrates, the polar metabolites being more easily conjugated or excreted. Several experiments have demonstrated that the halogenated polycyclics induce hepatic monooxygenases responsible for some steroid oxygenations, thereby altering the clearance of the steroid (Kupfer, 1975).

Orberg and Kihlstrom (1973), as well as others (Linder et al., 1974) have demonstrated that treatment with DDT or PCB's increases the length of the estrus cycle, and decreases the frequency of implantation in the sexually mature mouse. As expected, increasing the clearance of steroids, whether exogenous or endogenous, limits their biological activity. A direct relationship between monooxygenase activity and inhibition of uterine weight response to estrone has been demonstrated (Welch et al., 1971). Similar alterations in androgen effects have been observed in PCB-treated male rats (Derr and Dekker, 1979), and chickens (Nowicki and Norman, 1972). Other inducers of microsomal monooxygenases alter the estrogen or androgen activity of endogenous or exogenous steroids (Fahim et al., 1968, 1970). Both estrogen agonist and monooxygenase induction activities of the halogenated polycyclics represent potential mechanisms for reproductive toxicity in humans.

Indirect evidence suggests that halogenated polycyclics can induce monooxygenase activities in humans (Poland et al., 1970; Kolmodin et al., 1969), raising the possibility of similar mechanisms of fertility impairment in humans. Reproductive dysfunction has been observed in rhesus monkeys treated with halogenated polycyclics (Allen et al., 1979), as well as oocyte destruction by hexachlorobenzene (Iatropoulos et al., 1976).

Hexachlorophene impairs spermatogenesis, mating behavior, and prostatic development in male rats, but appears to have no effect on reproduction in female rats (Gellert et al., 1978; Thorpe, 1967, 1969).

The halogenated polycyclic hydrocarbons also have varying degrees of fetal toxicity and teratogenicity (Lucier and McDaniel, 1979; Kimbrough, 1974). An unfortunate accidental contamination of rice oil in Japan with several halogenated polycyclic hydrocarbons demonstrated that if these compounds are ingested, they can cross the placenta and produce human fetal toxicity. Menstrual cycle abnormalities were also noted in women ingesting the contaminated rice oil (Kimbrough, 1974).

Dibromochloropropane

Dibromochloropropane (DBCP) is a soil fumigant which was used until recently as a nematocide. Early toxicological studies in rats, rabbits, guinea pigs, and monkeys demonstrated that DBCP treatment produced severe testicular atrophy and degeneration (Torkelson et al., 1961). In the mid-1970's a group of men working in a pesticide-formulating factory in California became aware that many of them are infertile. Subsequent investigation of these workers confirmed that there was a high rate of infertility, without changes in libido, among these men (Whorton et al., 1977). Examination of these workers demonstrated an inverse relationship between length of occupational exposure to DBCP and sperm count, and a direct relationship between length of exposure and abnormal testicular morphology (Marshall et al., 1978). Although gonadotropins were decreased in these men, no changes in testosterone were observed, consistent with the observed persistence of libido.

DBCP is probably not directly toxic, but requires metabolism to a reactive intermediate before toxicity occurs. Recent studies have demonstrated that DBCP reduces or destroys hepatic monooxygenases (Moody et al., 1980). Since these enzymes are involved in both steroid production and clearance, this could account for the decrease in gonadotropins without change in the levels of testosterone. Recent studies have also demonstrated that DBCP produces dominant lethal mutations in male rats (Teramoto et al., 1980).

DBCP is interesting, demonstrating similar reproductive toxicity in humans and experimental animals. Moreover, humans appear more sensitive. Studies by Torkelson et al. (1961) referred to earlier suggested that the threshold for testicular toxicity was greater than 1 ppm. Air surveys in the pesticide-formulating factory demonstrated levels below 1 ppm, suggesting that the threshold in humans is below that for rodents and non-human primates.

Although gonadal toxicity in experimental animals does not indicate that human susceptibility will occur, it must serve as a warning that toxicity is possible. In the example given above, it appears that no attempt was made to determine if the occupational exposure to DBCP altered testicular function, with the workers themselves recognizing the gonadal toxicity.

Polycyclic Aromatic Hydrocarbons

The polycyclic aromatic hydrocarbons (PAH) are ubiquitous environmental pollutants produced by combustion of fossil fuels and contained in: automobile exhaust, smoke stack emissions, and cigarette smoke (NAS Committee, 1972). Although these compounds have long been known to be toxic and carcinogenic, recent studies have also demonstrated reproductive toxicity (Mattison, 1980; Mattison and Thorgeirsson, 1979; Wyrobeck and Bruce, 1975).

Several PAH's have been demonstrated to destroy oocytes in weanling and sexually mature rats and mice (Mattison, 1979). Treatment of a pregnant female will also destroy oocytes in an in utero female fetus (Felton et al., 1978). The mechanism of ac-

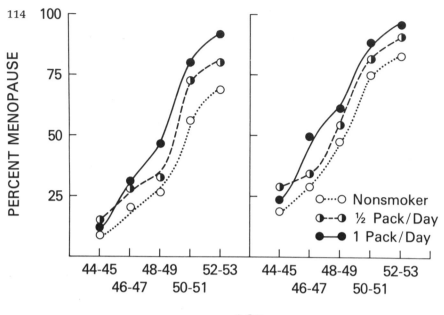

Fig. 3. Effects of cigarette smoking on the age of menopause in women in America (left panel), and women in seven European countries (right panel). (Adapted from the data of Jick et al., 1977.)

tion is thought to depend on metabolism of the parent PAH to a chemically reactive intermediate which binds covalently to cellular macromolecules destroying the oocytes (Mattison et al., 1979; Mattison and Thorgeirsson, 1979). The effect of oocyte destruction is to produce premature ovarian failure in the treated animals. Recent experiments have also suggested that certain PAH's can alter the ability of oocytes to complete meiosis (Basler and Rohrborn, 1976), suggesting another mechanism for reproductive failure after ovulation.

Susceptibility of human or non-human primates to oocyte destruction by PAH is not known. However, it has been demonstrated that smoking produces a dose-dependent decrease in the age of spontaneous menopause (Fig. 3). Women smoking one or more packs of cigarettes per day have menopause approximately two years before non-smokers. Women smoking half a pack of cigarettes per day have a median age of menopause about one year before non-smokers (Jick et al., 1977; Daniell, 1976). It has been suggested that the effect of smoking on the age of menopause is due to oocyte destruction by PAH in cigarette smoke (Mattison and Thorgeirsson, 1978). Many studies have suggested that cigarette smoke and nicotine can impair reproduction and fetal development in experimental animals as well as humans (Coleman et al., 1979; The Health Consequences, 1980). It is not known if these adverse effects result from PAH's, nicotine, carbon monoxide, or protein pyrolysates (Sugimura et al., 1977), all known constituents of cigarette smoke.

Alkylating Agents

Alkylating agents are useful in both the chemical industry and therapeutics because of their chemical reactivity. In the chemical industry, they are used in a broad spectrum of synthetic reactions, and in therapeutics they are useful in treating neoplastic and some non-neoplastic diseases. The alkylating agents are also interesting because they represent known reproductive toxins used in humans, permitting comparison of species differences in toxicity, detoxification, and repair.

One of the first alkylating agents used therapeutically, busulfan, is known to produce gonadal failure in humans and experimental animals (Hemsworth and Jackson, 1962, 1963; Jackson et al., 1959; Heller et al., 1964).

The alkylating agent to be considered here is the widely used drug, cyclophosphamide. High-dose intermittent therapy for neoplastic disease with cyclophosphamide alone or in combination with other drugs destroys oocytes in an age and dose-dependent manner (Koyama et al., 1977; Sirus et al., 1976; Sobrinho et al., 1971). Other antitumor drugs also impair fertility (Chapman et al., 1979a,b; Sieber and Adamson, 1975; Himelstein-Braw et al., 1977, 1978). Similar reproductive dysfunction is also seen in women treated with chronic oral cyclophosphamide for other diseases (Warne et al., 1973; Kumar et al., 1972).

Experiments in my laboratory in collaboration with Dr. Snorri S. Thorgeirsson of the National Cancer Institute have demonstrated a similar age and dose dependence for oocyte destruction in mice after treatment with cyclophosphamide as was observed in women. The results of these experiments suggest that age-dependent changes in pathways for detoxification of the reactive metabolite of cyclophosphamide account for age-dependent differences in sensitivity to oocyte destruction seen in both rodents and humans.

Gonadal dysfunction is also seen in males with neoplastic or non-neoplastic diseases treated with alkylating agents as well as other antineoplastic drugs (Hsu et al., 1979; Parra et al., 1978; Etteldorf et al., 1976; Jackson et al., 1959; Freeman-Narrod and Narrod, 1977; Kumar et al., 1972; Fairley et al., 1972; Lentz et al., 1977).

An interesting difference in age-dependent sensitivity for gonadal toxicity from cyclophosphamide exists between males and females. Young females are more sensitive to oocyte destruction than older females. In males, however, the young (prepubescent) animal is more resistant to testicular toxicity than the older male. This difference in sensitivity represents differences in both reproductive and toxicological mechanisms. The rate of spermatogenesis in the prepubertal testis is very low, and since spermatogenesis is sensitive to cyclophosphamide, suppression of sperm cell division will provide some degree of protection against toxicity, consistent with the observed age-dependent difference in testicular toxicity.

In the female, however, the most sensitive population appear to be the resting or small oocytes. As these are present throughout most of the life of the female in the same metabolic state, this cannot account for age-dependent differences in sensitivity. There is evidence, however, that the pathways for detoxification of the reactive metabolite(s) of cyclophosphamide change with age, and that these changes parallel the observed changes in sensitivity. Therefore, the opposite age-dependent changes in ovarian and testicular sensitivity to cyclophosphamide can be explained on the basis of an understanding of both reproductive biology and toxicology.

The mechanism of reproductive toxicity of cyclophosphamide results from metabolic activation of the parent compound and formation of reactive intermediates. Detoxification of reactive metabolites occurs through conjugation. Repair of resulting cellular damage after cyclophosphamide treatment requires replacement of damaged macromolecules and DNA repair.

In the testis, repopulation of seminiferous tubules will occur if spermatogonia remain after cessation of cyclophosphamide toxicity. In the ovary, however, since oogonia are not present after birth, oocyte destruction is permanent and irreplaceable. Cyclophosphamide has also been demonstrated to impair meiosis in rodent oocytes (Rohrborn and Hansmann, 1971).

Industrial exposure to alkylating agents or plasticizers (Oishi and Hiraga, 1979) may alter fertility in males or females. It is important, therefore, to monitor both the ambient levels of these industrial compounds as well as the reproductive function in workers exposed to these agents.

Cadmium

Cadmium salts produce testicular necrosis and subsequent atrophy secondary to testicular vascular damage in rodents (Patanelli, 1975; Gunn and Gould, 1970; Johnson, 1977; Dixon et al., 1976; Parizek, 1960). Human males exposed to cadmium may not be as sensitive as rodents; however, reversible infertility was observed in a monkey treated with cadmium.

The ovary does not appear to be as sensitive as the testis to cadmium toxicity (Parizek et al., 1968). The placenta, however, is sensitive to vascular damage after treatment with cadmium, producing fetal effects resulting from placental insufficiency (Parizek, 1964).

Boron

Reports from the USSR have suggested that exposure to boron oxides may produce oligospermia and decreased libido (Krasovski et al., 1976). Lee et al. (1978) have explored the effects of the common boron oxide $Na_2B_4O_7$ on the testis of rats and found a dose-dependent germinal aplasia. Similar effects have been observed in dogs treated with borax (Weir and Fisher, 1972) and rats treated with boron-containing tranquilizer (Truhant et al., 1964). Although the effects of boron on the testis were reversible at the lower doses used, at higher doses permanent azospermia resulted (Lee et al., 1978; Dixon et al., 1976). The mechanism and species susceptibility are unknown.

Summary

Successful reproduction, which is of crucial importance for all animals, depends upon the genetic, anatomic and endocrine integrity of the reproductive tract and gametes. I have briefly explored the mechanisms of reproduction toxicity and some selected reproductive toxins in this chapter, but I have by no means discussed all of the known or suspected reproductive toxins. The compounds chosen illustrate the multiple modes and sites of action available to reproductive toxins in both the male and female.

Because of the cryptic and periodic nature of human reproduction, other drugs or environmental xenobiotic compounds may currently be interfering with human or domestic animal reproduction, but remain undetected. The physician, in caring for his or her patients, must be alert to the possibility that a drug or occupational or environmental exposure may be jeopardizing their fertility.

References and Recommended Reading

1. Anderson, RA, Willis, BR, Oswald, C, Reddy, JM, Beyler, SA, Zaneveld, LJD: Hormonal imbalance and alterations in testicular morphology induced by chronic ingestion of ethanol. Biochem Pharmacol (In Press)

2. Aitio, A: Conjugation reactions in drug biotransformation. Elsevier, New York, 1978.

3. Akiyama, K, Ohi, G, Fugitani, K, Yagu, H, Ogino, M, Kawana T: Polychlorinated biphenyl residues in maternal and cord blood in Tokyo metropolitan area. Bull Environ Contam Toxicol 14:588, 1975.

4. Allen, JR, Barsotti, DA, Lambrecht, LK, Van Miller, JP: Reproductive effects of halogenated aromatic hydrocarbons on nonhuman primates. Ann NY Acad Sci 320:419, 1979.

5. Barnes, AB, Colton, T, Gundersen, J, Noller, KL, Tilley, BC, Strama, T, Townsend, DE, Hatab, P, O'Brain, PC: Fertility and outcome of pregnancy in women exposed in utero to diethylstilbestrol. N Engl J Med 302:609, 1980.

6. Basler, A, Rohrborn, G: Chromosome aberrations in oocytes of NMRI mice and bone marrow cells of Chinese hamsters induced with 3,4-benzpyrene mutation. Res 38:327, 1976.

7. Bibbo, M, Al-Nageeb, M, Baccarini, I, Gill, W, Newton, M, Sleeper, K, Sonek, M, Weid, GL: Follow-up study of male and female offspring of DES-treated mothers. A preliminary report. J Reprod Med 15:29, 1975.

8. Bibbo, M, Gill, WB, Azizi, F, Blaigh, R, Fang, VS, Rosenfield, RL, Schumacher, GF, Sleeper, K, Sonek, M, Weid, GL: Follow-up study of male and female offspring of DES-exposed mothers. Obstet Gyn 49:1, 1977.

9. Bitman, J, Cecil, HC: Estrogenic activity of DDT analogs and polychlorinated biphenyls. J Agr Food Chem 18:1108, 1970.

10. Blackburn, GM, Thompson, MH, King, HWS: Binding of diethylstilbestrol to deoxyribonucleic acid by rat liver microsomal fractions in vitro and in mouse foetal cells in culture. Biochem J 158:643, 1976.

11. Bourne, JP: A zodiac study of infertility: is season of birth associated with dysfunctions in ovulation? Department of Maternal and Child Health. The Johns Hopkins University School of Hygiene and Public Health, May, 1974.

12. Boylan, ES: Morphological and functional consequences of prenatal exposure to diethylstilbestrol in the rat. Biol Reprod 19:854, 1978.

13. Casarett, LJ, Doull, J (Eds.) Toxicology. The Basic Science of Poisons. Macmillan, New York, 1975.

14. Chapman, RM, Sutcliffe, SB, Malpas, JS: Cytotoxic-induced ovarian failure in women with Hodgkin's disease. I. Hormone function. JAMA 242:1877, 1979a.

15. Chapman, RM, Sutcliffe, SB, Malpas, JS: Cytotoxic-induced ovarian failure in women with Hodgkins disease. II. Effects on sexual function. JAMA 242:1882, 1979b.

16. Coleman, S, Pitrow, PT, Rinehart, W: Tobacco hazards to health and human reproduction. Population Reports. Issues in World Health Series L, No. 1, 1979.

17. Committee on biological effect of atmospheric pollutants. Particulate polycyclic organic matter. National Academy of Sciences, Washington, DC, 1972.

18. Cuhna, GR: Epithelial-stromal interactions in the development of the urogenital tract. Int Rev Cytol 47:137-194, 1976.

19. Daniell, HW: Osteoporosis of the slender smoker. Arch Intern Med 136:298, 1976.

20. Derr, SK, Dekker, J: Alterations of androgenicity in rats exposed to PCB's (Aroclor. 1254). Bull Environ Contam Toxicol 21:43, 1979.

21. Dieckmann, WJ, Davis, ME, Rynkiewicz, SM, Pottinger, RE: Does the administration of diethylstilbestrol during pregnancy have therapeutic value. Amer J Obstet Gynec 66:1062, 1953.

22. Dixon, RL: Symposium on Target Organ Toxicity: Gonads (Reproductive and Genetic Toxicity). Environ Health Perspect 24:1, 1978.

23. Dixon, RL, Lee, IP, Sherins, RJ: Methods to assess reproductive effects of environmental chemicals: Studies of cadmium and boron administered orally. Environ Hlth Perspect 13:59, 1976.

24. Dixon, RL, Lee, IP: Pharmacokinetic and adaptation factors involved in testicular toxicity. Federation Proc 39:66, 1980.

25. Doull, J: Factors influencing toxicology. In Toxicology. The Basic Science of Poisons. (Eds., LJ Caserett and J Doull) Macmillan, New York, 1975.

26. Etteldorf, JN, West, CD, Pitcock, JA, Williams, DL: Gonadal function, testicular histology, and meiosis following cyclophosphamide therapy in patients with nephrotic syndrome. J Pediatr 88:206, 1976.

27. Eversmann, T, Landfraf, R, Londong, W, Von Werder, K: Effect of cimetidine on prolactin-secretion and glucose tolerance in men. Horm Metab Res 11:412, 1979.

28. Fahim, MS, Dement, DG, Hall, DG, Fahim, Z: Induced alterations in hepatic metabolism of androgens in the rat. Amer J Obstet Gynec 107:1085, 1970.

29. Fahim, MS, King, TM, Hall, DG: Induced alterations in the biologic activity of estrogen. Amer J Obstet Gynecol 100:171, 1968.

30. Fairley, KF, Barrie, JU, Johnson, W: Sterility and testicular atrophy related to cyclophosphamide therapy. Lancet 1:568, 1972.

31. Felton, JS, Kwan, TC, Wuebbles, BJ, Dobson, RL: Genetic differences in polycyclic aromatic hydrocarbon metabolism and their effects on oocyte killing in developing mice. In Developmental Toxicology of Energy Related Pollutants. (DD Mahlum, MR, Sikov, PL Hackett, FD Andrew, Eds.) D.O.E. Symposium Series 47:1526, 1978.

32. Fleischer, S, Packer, L (Eds.): Biomembranes, Part C: Biological oxidations, microsomal, cytochrome P-450, and other hemoprotein systems. In Methods in Enzymology, Vol. 52. Academic Press, New York, 1978.

33. Forsberg, JG: An estradiol mitotic rate inhibiting effect in the mullerian epithelium in neonatal mice. J Exp Zool 175:369, 1970.

34. Forsberg, JG: Estrogen, vaginal cancer, and vaginal development. Amer J Obstet Gynec 113:83, 1972.

35. Forsberg, JG: The development of atypical epithelium in the mouse uterine cervix and vaginal fornix after neonatal oestradiol treatment. Brit J Exp Path 50:187, 1969.

36. Freeman-Narrod, M, Narrod, SA: Chronic toxicity of methotrexate in mice. J Natl Cancer Inst 58:735, 1977.

37. Gellert, RJ, Heinrichs, WL, Swerdloff, RS: DDT homologues: estrogen-like effects on the vagina, uterus and pituitary of the rat. Endocrinology 91:1095, 1972.

120

38. Gellert, RJ, Heinrichs, WL, Swerdloff, R: Effects of neonatally administered DDT homologs on reproductive function in male and female rats. Neuroendocrinology 16:84, 1974.

39. Gellert, RJ, Heinrichs, WL: Effects of DDT homologs administered to female rats during the perinatal period. Biol Neonate 26:283, 1975.

40. Gellert, RJ, Wallace, CA, Weismeier, EM, Shuman, RM: Topical exposure of neonates to hexachlorophene: longstanding effects on mating behavior and prostatic development in rats. Toxicol Appl Pharmacol 43:339, 1978.

41. Gellert, RJ: Uterotrophic activity of polychlorinated biphenyls (PCB) and induction of precocious reproductive aging in neonatally treated female rats. Environ Res 16:123, 1978.

42. Generoso, WM, Cain, KT, Krishna, M, Huff, S: Genetic lesions induced by chemicals in spermatozoa and spermatids of mice are repaired in the egg. Proc Natl Acad Sci U.S.A. 76:435, 1979.

43. Githens, JH, Rosenkrantz, JG, Tunnock, SM: Teratogenic effects of azathioprine (Imuran). J Pediatr 66:959, 1965.

44. Gomes, WR: Chemical agents affecting testicular function and male fertility. In The Testis, Vol. III (Eds., AD Johnson, WR Gomes, and NL Vandemark) Academic Press, New York, 1970, p. 483.

45. Gorski, RA: Gonadal hormones and the perinatal development of neuroendocrine function. In Frontiers in Neuroendocrinology (Eds., C Martini, WF Ganong) Oxford University Press, New York, 1971, p. 237.

46. Gross, A, Fein, A, Serr, DM, Nebel, L: The effect of Imuran on implantation and early embryonic development in rats. Obstet Gynec 50:713, 1977.

47. Gunn, SA, Gould, TC: Cadmium and other mineral elements. In The Testis, Vol. III (Eds., AD Johnson, WR Gomes, NL Vandemark) Academic Press, New york, 1970, p. 377.

48. Hall, WH: Breast changes in males on cimetidine. N Engl J Med 295:841, 1976.

49. Haney, AF, Hammond, CB, Soules, MR, Creasman, WT: Diethylstilbestrol-induced upper genital tract abnormalities. Fertil Steril 31:142, 1979.

50. Harrington, JM, Stein, GF, Rivera, RO, deMorales, AV: Occupational hazards of formulating oral contraceptives—A survey of plant employees. Arch Environ Health 33:12, 1978.

51. Heidelberger, C: Chemical carcinogenesis. Ann Rev Biochem 44:79, 1975.

52. Heinrichs, WL, Gellert, RJ, Bakke, JL, Lawrence, NL: DDT administered to neonatal rats induces persistent estrus syndrome. Science 173:642, 1971.

53. Heller, RH, Jones, HW, Blanchard, M: Production of ovarian dysgenesis in the rat and human by busulfan. Amer J Obstet Gynec 89:414, 1964.

54. Hemsworth, BN, Jackson, H: Effect of busulfan on the developing gonad of the male rat. J Reprod Fertil 5:187, 1962.

55. Hemsworth, BN, Jackson, H: Effect of busulfan on the developing ovary in the rat. J Reprod Fertil 6:229, 1963.

56. Herbst, AL, Hubby, NM, Blough, RR, Azizi, F: A comparison of pregnancy experience in DES-exposed and DES-unexposed daughters. J Reprod Med 24:62, 1980.

57. Herbst, AL, Ulfelder, H, Poskanser, DC: Adenocarcinoma of the vagina. Association of maternal stilbestrol therapy with tumor appearance in young women. N Engl J Med 284:878, 1971.

58. Himelstein-Braw, R, Peters, H, Faber, M: Influence of irradiation and chemotherapy on the ovaries of children with abdominal tumors. Brit J Cancer 36:269, 1977.

59. Himelstein-Braw, R, Peters, H, Faber, M: Morphological appearance of the ovaries of leukemic children. Brit J Cancer 38:82, 1978.

60. Hinckers, HJ: The influences of alcohol on the fetus. J Perinat Med 6:3, 1978.

61. Hsu, AC, Folami, AO, Bain, J, Rance, CP: Gonadal function in males treated with cyclophosphamide for nephrotic syndrome. Fertil Steril 31:173, 1979.

62. Iatropoulos, MJ, Hobson, W, Knauf, V, Adams, HP: Morphological effects of hexachlorobenzene toxicity in female rhesus monkeys. Toxicol Appl Pharmacol 37:433, 1976.

63. Jackson, H, Fox, BW, Craig, AW: The effect of alkylating agents on male rat fertility. Brit J Pharmacol 14:149, 1959.

64. Jick, H, Porter, J, Morrison, AS: Relation between smoking and age of natural menopause. Lancet 1:1354, 1977.

65. Johnson, AD: The influence of cadmium on the testis. In The Testis, Vol. IV (Eds., AD Johnson and WR Gomes) Academic Press, New York, 1977, p. 565.

66. Jones, KL, Smith, DW: The Fetal Alcohol Syndrome. Teratology 12:1, 1975.

67. Kaufman, RH, Binder, GL, Gray, PM, Adam, E: Upper genital tract changes associated with exposure in utero to diethylstilbestrol. Am J Obstet Gynec 128:51, 1977.

68. Kimbrough, RD: The toxicity of polychlorinated polycyclic compounds and related chemicals. Crit Rev Toxicol 2:445, 1974.

69. Kolmodin, B, Azarnoff, DL, Sjoqvist, F: Effect of environmental factors on drug metabolism: decreased plasma half-life of antipyrine in workers exposed to chlorinated hydrocarbon insecticides. Clin Pharm Therap 10:638, 1969.

70. Korach, KS, Metzler, M, McLachlan, JA: Diethylstilbestrol metabolites and analogs. New probes for the study of hormone action. J Biol Chem 254:8963, 1979.

71. Koyama, H, Wada, T, Nishizawa, Y, Iwanaga, T, Aoki, Y, Terasawa, T, Kosaki, G, Yamamoto, T, Wasa, A: Cyclophosphamide-induced ovarian failure and its therapeutic significance in patients with breast cancer. Cancer 39:1403, 1977.

72. Krasovski, GN, Varshavskaya, SP, Borisova, AF: Toxic and gonadotropic effects of cadmium and boron relative to standards for these substances in drinking water. Environ Health Perspect 13:69, 1976.

73. Kumar, R, Biggart, JD, McEvoy, J, McGeown, MG: Cyclophosphamide and reproductive function. Lancet 1:1212, 1972.

74. Kupfer, D: Effects of pesticides and related compounds on steroid metabolism and function. Crit Rev Toxicol 4:83, 1975.

75. Lee, IP, Dixon, RL: Factors influencing reproductive and genetic toxic effects on male gonads. Environ Health Perspect 24:117, 1978.

76. Lee, IP, Sherins, RJ, Dixon, RL: Evidence for induction of germinal aplasia in male rats by environmental exposure to boron. Toxicol Appl Pharmacol 45:577, 1978.

77. Lehmann, AR, Bridges, BA: DNA repair. Essays in Biochemistry. 13:71, 1977.

78. Lentz, RD, Bergstein, J, Steftes, MW, Brown, DR, Prem, K, Michael, AF, Vernier, RL: Postpubertal evaluation of gonadal function following cyclophosphamide therapy before and during puberty. J Pediatr 91:385, 1977.

79. Levi, AJ, Fisher, AM, Hughes, L, Hendry, WF: Male infertility due to sulphasalazine. Lancet 2:276, 1979.

80. Linder, RE, Gaines, TB, Kimbrough, RD: The effect of polychlorinated biphenyls on rat reproduction. Fd Cosmet Toxicol 12:63, 1974.

81. Lloyd, CW, Williams, RH: Endocrine changes associated with Laennec's cirrhosis of the liver. Am J Med 4:315, 1948.

82. Lucier, GW, Lee, IP, Dixon, RL: Effects of environmental agents on male reproduction. In The Testis, Vol. III (Eds., AD Johnson and WR Gomes) Academic Press, New York, 1977, p. 577.

83. Lucier, GW, McDaniel, OS: Developmental toxicology of the halogenated aromatics: Effects on enzyme development. Ann NY Acad Sci 320:449, 1979.

84. Marshall, S, Whorton, D, Krauss, RM, Palmer, WS: Effect of pesticides on testicular function. Urology 11:257, 1978.

85. Mattison, DR: Difference in sensitivity of rat and mouse primordial oocyte to destruction by polycyclic aromatic hydrocarbons. Chem Biol Interactions 28:133, 1979.

86. Mattison, DR: How xenobiotic compounds can destroy oocytes. Contemporary OB/GYN 15:157, 1980.

87. Mattison, DR: Morphology of oocyte and follicle destruction by polycyclic aromatic hydrocarbons in mice. Toxicol Appl Pharmac 53:249, 1980.

88. Mattison, DR., Shiromzu, K, Pendergrass, JA, Thorgeirsson, SS: Ontogeny of ovarian glutathione and sensitivity to primordial oocyte destruction by cyclophosphamide. (In preparation.)

89. Mattison, DR, Thorgeirsson, SS: Gonadal aryl hydrocarbon hydroxylase in rats and mice. Cancer Res 38:1368, 1978.

90. Mattison, DR, Thorgeirsson, SS: Ovarian aryl hydrocarbon hydroxylase activity and primordial oocyte toxicity of polycyclic aromatic hydrocarbon in mice. Cancer Res 39:3471, 1979.

91. Mattison, DR, Thorgeirsson, SS: Smoking and industrial pollution, and their effects on menopause and ovarian cancer. Lancet 1:187, 1978.

92. Mattison, DR, West, DM, Menard, RA: Differences in benzo(a) pyrene metabolic profile in rat and mouse ovary. Biochem Pharm 28:2101, 1979.

93. McLachlan, JA, Newbold, RR, Bullock, B: Reproductive tract lesions in male mice exposed prenatally to diethylstilbestrol. Science 190:991, 1975.

94. Metzler, M: Metabolic activation of carcinogenic diethylstilbestrol in rodents and humans. J Toxicol Environ Health Suppl 1:21, 1976.

95. Metzler, M, McLachlan, JA: Peroxidase-mediated oxidation, a possible pathway for metabolic activation of diethylstilbestrol. Biochem Biophys Res Commun 85:874, 1978.

96. Moody, DE, Head, B, Smuckler, EA: Reduction in hepatic microsomal cytochromes P-450 and b5 in rats exposed to 1,2-dibromo-3-chloropropane and carbon tetrachloride: Enhancement of effect by pretreatment with phenobarbital. J Environ Path Toxicol 3:177, 1980.

97. Mukhtar, H, Philpot, RM, Bend, JR: The postnatal development of micro-somal epoxide hydrose, cytosolic glutathione-S-transferase, and mitochon-drial and microsomal cytochrome P-450 in adrenals and ovaries of female rats. Drug Metab Dispos 6:577, 1978.

98. Nowicki, HG, Norman, AW: Enhanced hepatic metabolism of testoster-one 4-androstene-3,17-dione, and estradiol-17β in chickens pretreated with DDT or PCB. Steroids 19:85, 1972.

99. Oesch, F: Mammalian epoxide hydrase: inducible enzymes catalysing the inactivation of carcinogenic and cytotoxic metabolic derived from aro-matic and olefinic compounds. Xenobiotica 3:305, 1972.

100. Oishi, S, Hiraga, K: Effect of phthalic acid esters on gonadal function in male rats. Bull Environ Contam Toxicol 21:65, 1979.

101. O'Leary, JA, Davies, JE, Edmundson, WF, Reich, GA: Transplacental passage of pesticides. Amer J Obstet Gynec 107:65, 1970.

102. Orberg, J, Kihlstrom, JE: Effects of long-term feeding of polychlorinated biphenyls (PCB, Clophen A 60) on the length of the oestrous cycle and on the frequency of implanted ova in the mouse. Environ Res 6:176, 1973.

103. Ouellette, EM, Rosett, HL, Rosman, NP, Weiner, L: Adverse effects on off-spring of maternal alcohol abuse during pregnancy. N Engl J Med 297:528, 1977.

104. Parizek, J: Sterilization of the male by cadmium salts. J Reprod Fert 1:294, 1960.

105. Parizek, J: Vascular changes at sites of oestrogen biosynthesis produced by parenteral injection of cadmium salts: the destruction of the placenta by cadmium salts. J Reprod Fertil 7:263, 1964.

106. Parizek, J, Ostadalova, I, Benes, I, Pitha, J: The effect of a subcutaneous injection of cadmium salts on the ovaries of adult rats in persistent oestrus. J Reprod Fertil 17:559, 1968.

107. Parra, A, Santos, D, Cervantes, C, Sojo, I, Carranzo, A, Cortes-Gallegos, V: Plasma gonadotropins and gonadal steroids in children treated with cyclo-phosphamide. J Pediatr 92:117, 1978.

108. Patanelli, DJ: Suppression of fertility in the male. In Handbook of Phys-iology. Section 7: Endocrinology, Vol. 5, The Male Reproductive System. (Eds. DW Hamilton and RO Greep, p. 245) American Physiological Society, Wash-ington, DC, 1975.

109. Pedersen, RA, Manigia, F: Ultraviolet light-induced unscheduled DNA synthesis by resting and growing mouse oocytes. Mutat Res 49:425, 1978.

110. Poland, A, Smith, D, Kuntzman, R, Jacobson, M, Conney, AH: Effect of intensive occupational exposure to DDT on phenylbutazone and cortisol me-tabolism in human subjects. Clin Pharm Therap 11:724, 1970.

111. Polishuk, LW, Wasserman, M, Wasserman, D, Groner, Y, Lazarovici, S, Tomatis, L: Effects of pregnancy on storage of organochlorine insecticides. Arch Environ Health 20:215, 1970.

112. Reimers, TJ, Sluss, PM: 6-Mercaptopurine treatment of pregnant mice: effects on second and third generations. Science 201:65, 1978.

113. Reimers, TJ, Sluss, PM, Goodwin, J, Seidel, GE: Bi-generational effects of 6-mercaptopurine on reproduction in mice. Biol Reprod 22:367, 1980.

114. Rohrborn, G, Hansmann, I: Induced chromosome aberrations in un-fertilized oocytes of mice. Humangenetik 13:184, 1971.

115. Rudiger, HW, Haenisch, F, Metzler, M, Oesch, F, Glatt, HR: Metabolites of diethylstilbestrol induce sister chromatid exchange in cultured human fibroblasts. Nature 281:392, 1979.

116. Schmidt, G, Fowler, WC, Talbert, LM, Edelman, DA: Reproductive history of women exposed to diethylstilbestrol in utero. Fert Steril 33:21, 1980.

117. Shepard, TH: Catalog of Teratogenic Agents. The Johns Hopkins University Press, Baltimore, 2nd Edition, 1976.

118. Sieber, SM, Adamson, RH: Toxicity of antineoplastic agents in man: Chromosomal aberrations, antifertility effects, congenital malformations and carcinogenic potential. Adv Cancer Res 22:57, 1975.

119. Sims, P, Grover, PL: Epoxides in polycyclic aromatic hydrocarbon metabolism and carcinogenesis. Adv Cancer Res 20:165, 1974.

120. Sirus, ES, Leventhal, BG, Vaitukaitis, JL: Effects of childhood leukemia and chemotherapy on puberty and reproductive function in girls. N Engl J Med 294:1143, 1976.

121. Smith, OW: Diethylstilbestrol in the prevention and treatment of complications of pregnancy. Am J Obstet Gynec 56:821, 1948.

122. Sobrinho, LG, Levine, RA, DeConti, RC: Amenorrhea in patients with Hodgkin's disease treated with antineoplastic agents. Amer J Obstet Gynec 109:135, 1971.

123. Sugimura, T, Nagao, M, Kawachi, T et al.: Mutagen-carcinogens in food with special reference to highly mutagenic pyrolytic products in broiled foods. In Origins of Human Cancer (Eds., HH Hiatt, JD Watson, AJ Winstein) Cold Spring Harbor Laboratory, 1977, p. 1561.

124. Teramoto, S, Saito, R, Aoyama, H, Shirasu, Y: Dominant lethal mutation induced in male rats by 1,2-dibromo-3-chloropropane (DBCP). Mutat Res 77:71, 1980.

125. The Health Consequences of Smoking for Women. A Report of the Surgeon General. U.S. Department of H.E.W., Public Health Service, 1980.

126. Thorpe, E: Some pathological effects of hexachlorophene in the rat. J Comp Pathol 77:137, 1967.

127. Thorpe, E: Some toxic effects of hexachlorophene in sheep. J Comp Pathol 79:167, 1969.

128. Torkelson, TR, Sadek, SE, Rowe, VK, Kodama, JK, Anderson, HH, Loquvam, GS, Hine, CH: Toxicologic investigation of 1,2-dibromo-3-chloropropane. Toxicol Appl Pharm 3:545, 1961.

129. Toth, A: Male infertility due to sulphasalazine. Lancet 2:904, 1979b.

130. Toth, A: Reversible toxic effect of salicylazosulfapyridine on semen quality. Fertil Steril 31:538, 1979a.

131. Traub, AI, Thompson, W, Carville, J: Male infertility due to salphasalazine Lancet 2:639, 1979.

132. Truhant, R, Phu-Lich, H, Loisillier, F: Sur les effets de l'ingestin repetee de petites doses de derives du bore sur les fonctions de reproduction du rat. C.H.R. Acad Sci 258:5099, 1964.

133. Uldall, PR, Kerr, DNS, Tacchi, D: Sterility and cyclophosphamide. Lancet 1:693, 1972.

134. Van Thiel, DH, Gravaler, JS, Cobb, CF, Sherins, RJ, Lester, R: Alcohol-induced testicular atrophy in the adult male rat. Endocrinology 105:888, 1979a.

135. Van Thiel, DH, Gavaler, JS, Smith, WI, Paul, G: Hypothalamic-pitui-tary-gonadal dysfunction in men using cimetidine. N Engl J Med 300:1012, 1979b.

136. Vorherr, H, Messer, RH, Vorherr, UF, Jordan, SW, Kornfeld, M: Terato-genesis and carcinogenesis in rat offspring after transplacental and trans-mammary exposure to diethylstilbestrol. Biochem Pharmac 28:1865, 1979.

137. Warne, GL, Fairley, KF, Hobbs, JB, Martin, FIR: Cyclophosphamide in-duced ovarian failure. N Engl J Med 289:1159, 1973.

138. Weir, RJ, Fisher, RS, Toxicologic studies on borax and boric acid. Tox-icol Appl Pharmacol 23:351, 1972.

139. Welch, RM, Levin, W, Conney, AH: Estrogenic action of DDT and its analogs. Toxicol Appl Pharmacol 14:358, 1969.

140. Welch, RM, Levin, W, Kuntzman, Jacobson, M, Conney, AH: Effect of halogenated hydrocarbon insecticides on the metabolism and uterotropic ac-tion of estrogens in rats and mice. Toxicol Appl Pharmacol 19:234, 1971.

141. Whorton, D, Krauss, RM, Marshall, S, Milby, TH: Infertility in male pes-ticide workers. Lancet 2:1259, 1977.

142. Winters, SJ, Banks, JL, Loriaux, DL: Cimetidine is an antiandrogen in the rat. Gastroenterology 76:504, 1979.

143. Wolf, MM: Impotence on cimetidine treatment. N Engl J Med 300:94, 1979.

144. Wong, TW, Hruban, Z: Testicular degeneration and necrosis induced by chlorcyclizine. Lab Invest 26:278, 1972.

145. Woolley, DE, Talens, GM: Distribution of DDT, DDD, and DDE in tis-sues of neonatal rats and in milk and other tissues of mother rats chronically exposed to DDT. Toxicol Appl Pharmacol 18:907, 1971.

146. Wyrobeck, AJ, Bruce, WR: Chemical induction of sperm abnormalities in mice. Proc Natl Acad Sci USA 72:4425, 1975.

5

LEGAL CONSIDERATIONS IN MEDICAL PRACTICE

Legal Considerations in Medical Practice with Reference to the Administration of Drugs in Pregnancy

ROGER SCOTT, J.D.

PROFESSIONAL RESPONSIBILITY

Standard of Care

It is a truism that any professional conduct carries with it professional responsibility. As applied to physicians, lack (or what may be misconceived as lack) of professional responsibility is generally referred to as "malpractice." The question of malpractice arises only when an injury or a "bad result" occurs. In such instances, several factors can enter in the deliberations to determine if, indeed, there was a lack of professional responsibility.

There is no requirement that a physician *guarantee* a "good result" when a medical service is performed, nor that he possess the extraordinary knowledge and ability enjoyed by only a few people of rare and uncommon endowments. In rendering this service, however, the physician is required to use his best judgment, reasonable care, and to exercise that reasonable degree of knowledge and skill possessed by similar professionals in the community. The latter is the physician's *medical community*

Mr. Scott is a practicing attorney in New York State, and a partner in the law firm of Scott, Sardano and Pomeranz.

and does not necessarily conform to political or geographical subdivisions. Specialists may establish their own standard of care and even raise the standards of their community. Although at present it is not required that a physician practice at a national or world standard of expertise—and there are no communities based on areas as large as a state for the purpose of determining the standards of care—the trend is to expand the boundaries of a physician's community. This trend is perhaps a result of improved communication. A physician may be required to acquire knowledge that might not have been available to him in past years. If the trend in information processing and communications continues, the future may well hold a requirement that physicians be held to the same standard without regard to the location of practice. State, national, or world standards may be in use in the foreseeable future. Department of Health, Education, and Welfare regulations are beginning to establish a minimum national standard in particular areas, such as educational research. In this chapter references are made to New York law. Differing views may occur in other states. The need to refer to the laws of the state in which a physician practices is strongly stressed.

In exercising his best judgment a physician is not responsible for a mere error in judgment, provided the course of action was reasonable as judged by community practice. Similarly, the rule of reasonable care does not require the exercise of the highest possible degree of care, but only that degree of care that a reasonably prudent physician would exercise under the same circumstances. Negligence may therefore be defined as a lack of "ordinary care."

There are several elements in the concept of negligence. The latter may arise from either the performance or the failure to perform a particular act or acts. The danger of injury must be foreseeable, i.e., probable, not merely possible. If a reasonably prudent physician could not foresee any injury as a result of his or her conduct, or if his or her conduct was reasonable in the light of what he or she could foresee, the physician is not negligent. Similarly, if the standard of care in the community does not include a particular knowledge, his lack of that knowledge would not be negligence. On the other hand, if a physician has the knowledge but refuses or fails to use it, that refusal or failure could be considered negligence. Although the acceptable standards of practice are properly the subject of testimony by expert witnesses, it is the jury who must decide what the standard is.

In making a determination, the jury is required to make that determination within the limits of the available testimony in that particular case. Because so many factors contribute to a jury's decision, it is generally not possible to use any particular case as an example. If those awards are within the scope of the evidence submitted, an Appellate Court will generally not overturn that verdict. The jury is the sole determiner of the facts in any particular case, and the court determines only the law of that particular case. Therefore, general rules cannot be drawn from the outcome of any particular case. Legal pronouncements, especially when made by Appellate Courts, can be relied upon as guidelines for proper conduct.

Concealment of Malpractice

The intentional concealment of an act of malpractice gives rise to a cause of action for fraud, providing the element of the *tort of deceit* can be established. In such cases it must be proven that the physician knew or should have known of the malpractice and the consequent injury to the patient; and thereafter knowingly made false material and factual misrepresentations with respect to the subject matter of the malpractice and the therapy appropriate to its cure; the traditional elements of the *tort of deceit* must be established and damages measured by the cost of cure or correction, provided that the condition caused by the malpractice could be corrected or alleviated. (If there is no available efficacious cure from which the patient is diverted by deceit, there will be nominal or no damages, but if it is established that the deceit prevented complete cure, then the damages will be greater, accordingly.) In addition, claims may be based upon the theory of a contract to produce a particular result, or to follow a particular method, or to produce a particular result within a specified period of time.

Informed Consent

It is essential to obtain the patient's informed consent before performing a medical service. In terms understandable by a reasonable person the patient should be informed of the reason for the medical procedure, what the risks to the patient's health or life may be in performing the medical procedure, what the risks may be if no procedure is performed, whether the procedure proposed is one that is ordinarily done under the same conditions, whether other or different procedures, if any, are used, the manner in which the alternative procedures are performed, and the nature and extent of the risks involved in the alternative procedures. The physician is required to give this information to the patient so that when the patient's consent is given, it is given with an awareness of the existing physical condition, the purpose and advantages that warrant being submitted to the procedure, the risks to his health or his life which the procedure may impose, the risks involved if no procedure is performed, and the available alternate procedures and the risks involved in those. It is no defense that the procedure which was performed was a medically sound procedure, since it is the patient's right to decide whether or not to consent to the procedure. The question is not what the patient would have decided, but what would a reasonably prudent person in the patient's circumstances, having sufficient knowledge of the material risks of, and alternatives to the medical procedure, have decided. If a physician gives a patient all of the facts required to be given, or if the information omitted would not have materially affected the patient's decision to submit to the procedure, then there is no liability on the part of the physician for failure to obtain informed consent.

Informed consent is required when the treatment involved is an invasion of the patient's physical integrity. Operating without informed consent is equivalent to operating without any consent at all and in addition, raises the issue of assault and battery. Failure to inform the patient of his or her condition under circumstances not involving an invasion of the patient's physical integrity is not a claim for lack of informed consent, and instead may be the basis for a claim for medical malpractice. The exact scope of the information to be imparted will vary with each individual case, and in some cases, the patient's mental and emotional condition may be a factor. In a particular case, concealing some of the possible consequences may be proper.

In New York there is a division of authority as to whether the standard by which to determine what information should be given to patients is to be measured by prevailing medical practice, or measured by the general standard of reasonableness. If it is to be measured by the prevailing medical practice, then expert witnesses would be required to establish the prevailing medical practice. If it is to be measured by the standard of reasonableness, it is a question for the jury as a question of fact. The general view is that the question of what, and under what circumstances the patient should be informed, is a question ultimately for determination by a jury as a question of fact. In that case, medical testimony may be appropriate but not required. In claims arising on or after July 1, 1975, expert testimony is required for a claimant-patient to recover on the theory of his lack of informed consent.

The issue of informed consent is also pertinent for institutional review boards when applied to educational research. The code of federal regulations require that the consent obtained be "legally effective." The consent obtained must be both free and knowing, and may not contain exculpatory language. It must include:

1) A fair explanation of the procedures to be followed and their purposes, including identification of any procedures which are experimental;

2) A description of any attendant discomforts and risks to be reasonably expected;

3) A description of any benefits to be reasonably expected;

4) A disclosure of any appropriate alternative procedures that might be advantageous for the subject;

5) An offer to answer any inquiries concerning the procedures;

6) An instruction that the person is free to withdraw his consent and discontinue participation in the project or activity at any time without prejudice to the subject.

A consent document that contains all of the above elements may also satisfy the informational component of informed consent required by the courts.

In New York State, as in several other states, there is currently a specific statutory provision concerning lack of informed consent. This statutory provision, Section 2805-d of the Public Health Law of the State of New York, provides:

1. Lack of informed consent means the failure of the person providing the professional treatment or diagnosis to disclose to the patient such alternatives thereto, and the reasonably foreseeable risks and benefits involved, as a reasonable medical practitioner under similar circumstances would have disclosed, in a manner permitting the patient to make a knowledgeable evaluation.

2. The right of action to recover for medical malpractice based on lack of informed consent is limited to those cases involving either

(a) non-emergency treatment, procedure, or surgery, or

(b) a diagnostic procedure which involved invasion or disruption of the integrity of the body.

3. For a cause of action therefore, it must also be established that a reasonably prudent person in the patient's position would not have undergone the treatment or diagnostic procedure if he had been fully informed, and that the lack of informed consent

is a proximate cause of the injury or condition for which recovery is sought.

4. It shall be a defense to any action for medical malpractice based upon an alleged failure to obtain such an informed consent that

(a) the risk not disclosed is too commonly known to warrant disclosure; or

(b) the patient assured the medical practitioner he would undergo the treatment, procedure, or diagnostic procedure regardless of the risk involved, or the patient assured the medical practitioner that he did not want to be informed of the matters to which he would be entitled to be informed; or

(c) consent by or on behalf of the patient was not reasonably possible; or

(d) the medical practitioner, after considering all of the attendant facts and circumstances, used reasonable discretion as to the manner and extent to which such alternatives or risks were disclosed to the patient because he reasonably believed that the manner and extent of such disclosure could reasonably be expected to adversely and substantially affect the patient's condition.

The Statute of Limitations

In almost all types of legal actions where a claim is made for damages, there is a specific period of time within which a lawsuit must be commenced. This provides a defendant with some protection against unlimited liability forever. The period of time within which a claim must be made is generally established by a law or statute, and is generally referred to as the "statute of limitations." It should be noted, however, that although the claim must be brought within the "statute of limitations," there is no necessity that it be brought within the lifetime of either the person bringing the claim or the defendant, i.e., a claim may be made against the physician's estate as long as it is within the "statute of limitations." The concept of the statute of limitations is quite simple in theory, but has been subject to so many statutory and decisional changes that in practice it has become quite complex. Each state sets its own statute of limitations for different types of lawsuits. In New York State, the statute of limitations for an adult claimant in a claim for professional malpractice is three years. The legislature in New York State, in response to the so-called "malpractice crisis," established a shorter period of limitation for claims accruing after July 1, 1975. For those claims, the statute of limitations is two years and six months. The differing period of limitations based on the date of the claim is not the only exception to a uniform, single "statute of limitations." There is the theory of the *tolling* or suspension of the statute of limitations. For instance, a claim based upon an injury to an infant based upon professional malpractice is tolled or suspended until the infant reaches the age of 18. Again, in New York, we have two different periods of time depending upon when the claim accrued. If a claim for an injury to an infant occurred prior to July 1, 1975, the statute of limitations is suspended until the infant reaches the age of 18. If the injury occurred after July 1, 1975, the claim for injury is tolled for 10 years from the date that the claim accrued. The applicable statute of limitations begins after the tolling has ended. For example, a claim brought on behalf of an infant for professional malpractice occurring on or after July 1, 1975 is tolled for 10 years and the infant has 2½ years thereafter to bring the claim. In order to determine the commencement of the statute of limitations, it must be determined when the claim begins. At first blush, this would seem to pose no difficulty, but there is a sharp division of authority among the different states on this item. Some states, such as New York, seem to have adopted the "first breath theory," while other states seem to have adopted the "discovery theory." The "first breath theory" provides that the claim begins when the actual act of malpractice has occurred, and does not depend upon when the injured party first discovers that he or she has been injured by an act of professional malpractice. The "discovery theory" provides that the statute of limitations does not begin to run until the injured person discovers that his or her injuries were caused by an act of malpractice, or discovers the actual injuries. In the case of a long-term injury, which does not show itself until many years after the act of professional malpractice, the statute of limitations could run before the evidence of the injury becomes apparent. In those situations, the injured party could not bring the claim, since he or she could not prove a compensable injury, and after the injury has become apparent so that it could be proved, the statute of limitations may have already expired. This theory is of particular importance in the case of the administration of drugs to a pregnant woman. If there is an act of malpractice, it probably occurs on the date that the drug is administered. In such cases, the statute of limitations could completely run before the effect of the drug is observable and provable. Extreme care should be taken when relying upon this theory of limitation, since it is not statutory, but is the result of court decisions. Court decisions, however straightforward they may appear, are always subject to later decisions which may alter or completely revoke prior court decisions.

To make matters more difficult in trying to determine when the statute of limitations has run, there are many exceptions. One exception is where the course of treatment, which includes the wrongful act complained of, has run continuously and is related to the original condition or complaint. In that case, the cause of action may accrue at the end of the treatment and not at the time of the initial act of professional malpractice. For such an exception to apply, the treatment must be performed continuously by the same physician who committed the act upon which the claim is based; and the period of continuous treatment by a single physician is not extended by further treatment provided by the patient's family physician or general practitioner, even if that further treatment is for the same condition or complaint. There are other exceptions. In New York State, there is an exception concerning foreign objects. If a foreign object is negligently left in the patient's body, the timeliness of the action depends upon when the injury occurred. If the foreign object results from an operation performed before July 1, 1975, a claim is timely commenced if it is made within three years of the discovery of the foreign object. If the operation was performed on or after July 1, 1975, the action is timely if brought within 2½ years after the operation, or within one year after the actual discovery of the foreign object, or within one year after discovery of facts which would reasonably lead to the discovery of a foreign object, whichever occurs first. For actions prior to July 1, 1975, a foreign object could include a chemical compound, but for claims arising after July 1, 1975, the New York State legislature specifically provided that a foreign object should not include a chemical compound, fixation device, or prosthetic aid or device.

Since the statute of limitations is established by each individual state, and is subject to frequent change both by the legislature and by the courts, it is necessary to determine in each case what the statute of limitations in that particular locality is for the time alleged in the complaint. Since the statute of limitations does not become critically important until after a claim is made, and since the statute of limitations may be researched with particularity after the nature of the claim is disclosed in the claim itself, and after the alleged date of professional malpractice has been stated, it is not as difficult to determine if the claim is being made timely in retrospect as it is to determine if it could be made timely for a prospective claim. It is therefore generally sufficient to understand that there is a statute of limitations, that the statute of limitations is not "written in stone," and that it is subject to numerous changes, variations and exceptions.

OBSTETRICAL CONSIDERATIONS
"Wrongful Life"

Relevant to the administration of drugs during pregnancy, and their possible effects on the fetus, is the question of the liability for what has been generally termed "wrongful life." Does a child have a cause of action against a physician for "wrongful life?" In New York, and many other states, if not all other states, the courts have rejected the claim for "wrongful life."

After a long history of dealing with this question, in an indication that the New York courts might have recognized a claim for "wrongful life," the highest court of the State of New York, recently in the case of *Becker v. Schwartz,* 46 N.Y.2d (1980) ruled that a complaint brought on behalf of an infant, alleging "wrongful life" (i.e., premised upon the birth of a fully intended but abnormal child for whom extraordinary care and treatment is required), claiming that the defendant physician negligently failed to inform the plaintiff's parents accurately of the risks involved in a pregnancy, that said negligence being instrumental either in the parents' decision to conceive or the parents' decision not to terminate the pregnancy, does not state a legally cognizable cause of action for two reasons: 1) it does not appear that the infant suffered any legally cognizable injury, as a child does not have a fundamental right to be born as a whole, functional human being; and 2) damages recoverable on behalf of an infant for "wrongful life" are not ascertainable, as damages are designed to place the injured party in a position he would have occupied but for the negligence of the defendant, and by the allegations of the complaint, but for the negligence of the defendant, the infant would not be in existence.

The Court of Appeals, as to the corollary action by the plaintiffs, indicated that a complaint brought by the parent of an infant, in their own right, alleging "wrongful life" (i.e., premised upon the birth of a fully intended but abnormal child for whom extraordinary care and treatment is required), claiming that defendant physicians failed to inform plaintiff's parents accurately of the risks involved in a pregnancy, said negligence being instrumental either in the parents' decision to conceive or the parents' decision not to terminate the pregnancy, does state a legally cognizable cause of action for the pecuniary damages suffered as a consequence of the birth as such damages are ascertainable; and the complaint alleges the existence of a duty flowing from defendants to plaintiffs and that the breach of that duty was a proximate cause of the damages. However, the court indicated that for policy reasons, parents were prevented from recovering damages for psychic or emotional harm alleged to have occurred as a consequence of the birth of an infant in an impaired state since the calculation of damages for such injuries is too speculative despite the breach of duty. Notwithstanding the birth of an afflicted child, and certainly dependent upon the extent of the affliction, parents may experience a love that even an abnormality cannot fully dampen which would be a necessary consideration in mitigation of any such damages.

This is an important case which should have an effect on many other states. In this case, it was the plaintiffs' contention that throughout the period during which Dolores Becker was under the care of defendants, the defendants never advised of the increased risk of Down's syndrome in children born to women over 35 years of age. It was also claimed that no advice was given as to the availability of an amniocentesis test to determine whether the fetus carried by Dolores Becker would be born afflicted with Down's syndrome. The plaintiffs commenced the action seeking damages on behalf of the infant for "wrongful life," and in their own right for various sums of money that they would be forced to expend for the long-term institutional care of the retarded child. Their complaint also sought damages for the emotional and physical injury suffered by Dolores Becker as a result of the birth of her child, as well as damages for the injury suffered by Arnold Becker occasioned by the loss of his wife's services and the medical expenses stemming from her treatment. The Court of Appeals heard a companion case at the same time involving a plaintiff, Hetty Park, who gave birth in June, 1969, to a baby afflicted with polycystic kidney disease who died only five hours after birth. Concerned with a possible recurrence of this disease in a child conceived in the future, Hetty Park and her husband, Steven Park, consulted the defendants, the obstetricians who treated Hetty Park during her first pregnancy, to determine the likelihood of this contingency. In response to the plaintiff's inquiry, the defendants are alleged to have informed the plaintiffs that inasmuch as polycystic kidney disease was not hereditary, the chances of their conceiving a second child afflicted with this disease were "practically nil." Based upon this information, the plaintiffs alleged that they exercised a conscious choice to seek conception of a second child. As a result, Hetty Park again became pregnant and gave birth in July of 1970 to a child who similarly suffered from polycystic kidney disease. Unlike their first child, however, plaintiffs' second child survived for two and one-half years before succumbing to the progressive disease. At that time, the plaintiffs alleged that contrary to the defendants' advice, polycystic kidney disease is in fact an inherited condition, and had they been correctly informed of the true risk of occurrence of this disease in a second child, they would not have chosen to conceive. The plaintiffs commenced this action seeking damages on behalf of the infant for "wrongful life," and in their own right, for the pecuniary expense they had borne for the care and treatment of their child until her death. The plaintiffs' complaint also sought damages for the emotional and physical injuries suffered by Hetty Park as a result of the birth of her child; damages for emotional injuries and expenses suffered by Steven Park; damages for the injury suffered by Steven Park occasioned by the loss of his wife's services; and damages on behalf of the plaintiffs as administrators of their child's estate for wrongful death.

In its decision, the Court took pains to emphasize that the Court was not deciding whether the plaintiffs should ultimately prevail in the litigation, but rather more narrowly, whether their complaints stated cognizable causes of action. The review of the Court, in its decision, was limited to an evaluation of the sufficiency of the plaintiff's complaints and for that reason, the Court assumed all of their allegations to be true. The Court went on to evaluate the prior history of claims for "wrongful life" and distinguished the claims for "wrongful birth" and "wrongful diagnosis." The Court distinguished between claims based on a wrongful conception, a failure to diagnose a pregnancy or an illegitimate birth, in which the essence of the wrong for which compensation was sought is the birth of a healthy and normal, albeit unplanned, child. The decision of the Court concerned the claims of the plaintiffs based upon the birth of a fully intended but abnormal child for whom extraordinary care and treatment is required. There was no claim that the defendant physicians' treatment of Dolores Becker and Hetty Park caused the abnormalities in their infants. The claim was only that *had the plain-*

tiffs been properly advised by the defendants of the risks of abnormality, their infants would never have been born.

The Court stated the broad principle of *medical malpractice,* requiring that a successful plaintiff must demonstrate the existence of a duty, the breach of which may be considered the proximate cause of the damages suffered by the injured party. The Court decided that the plaintiffs' complaint alleging claims on behalf of their infants whether denominated as claims for "wrongful life" or otherwise, failed to state legally cognizable causes of action. The Court determined that there is no precedent for recognition of any fundamental right of a child to be born as a whole, functional human being. The Court refused to determine whether it is better to never have been born at all than to have been born with even gross deficiencies, and deferred to a "very nearly uniform high value which the law and mankind has placed upon human life, rather than its absence." The Court found that there was no right of common law, nor was there any statutory enactment for judicial recognition of the birth of a defective child as an injury to the child. The Court also noted that the remedy afforded an injured party in negligence is designed to place that party in the position he would have occupied but for the negligence of the defendant. The Court of Appeals determined that the damages recoverable on behalf of an infant for wrongful life are limited to that which is necessary to restore the infant to the position he or she would have occupied were it not for the failure of the defendant to render advice to the infant's parents in a non-negligent manner. Since the claim alleged that had the defendant not been negligent, the infant's parents would have chosen not to conceive, or having conceived, to have terminated rather than to have carried the pregnancy to term, placing the infant in the position he or she would have occupied were it not for the failure of the defendant to render advice in a non-negligent manner would deprive the infant plaintiff of his or her very existence. The Court deferred to the legislature and stated that to recognize such a cause of action would require the creation of a hypothetical formula for the measurement of an infant's damages, best reserved for legislative rather than judicial attention. The Court therefore dismissed the plaintiffs' complaints insofar as they sought damages on behalf of their infants for wrongful life.

The legislature of any particular state could, of course, create a cause of action not known in the common law and not recognized by the Courts, and could create a cause of action for "wrongful life." Without statutory authority, the Courts of many states, as the Court of Appeals in New York State, have been reluctant to recognize or create a claim for "wrongful life." Courts have thereby avoided the difficult question of "being" vs. "non-being." It should be recognized, however, that the parents of a defective child have a cause of action based on negligence, if it can be proven that the physician's negligence *caused the condition*. The infant's parents may recover for traditionally "measurable" damages in their own right, accruing as a consequence of the birth of their defective infants.

There is a duty flowing from the involved physicians to the parents, and a breach of that duty could be the proximate cause of the birth of the defective infant. Unlike causes of actions brought on behalf of infants for wrongful life, causes of actions brought by parents, also founded essentially upon a theory of negligence or medical malpractice, do allege ascertainable damages. The damage may include the pecuniary expense which the parents have borne and which they may be required to continue to bear for the care and treatment of their infants which could be for the rest of the infant's life. Traditional tort theory would provide that but for the defendant physician's breach of his duty to advise the plaintiff parents, the plaintiff parents would not have been required to assume those obligations. Calculation of those damages necessary to make the parents whole in relation to the expenditures required to be made for the care and treatment of the injured infant, requires nothing extraordinary in being able to compute the value amount of damages. Such damages may include, in addition to the costs incurred in the care and treatment of the infant child, the expenses to the parents of such items as an unsuccessful sterilization followed by the birth of the child, the cost of the delivery of the child, the loss to the husband of consortium of the wife, etc. This is not to say that a plaintiff may recover for psychic or emotional harm to have been alleged as a consequence of the birth of a defective infant. The recovery of damages for such injuries is circumscribed by the decision of the New York State Court of Appeals in *Becker v. Schwartz*. The Court of Appeals reiterated the rule in a previous decision of *Howard v. Lecher* (42 NY2d 109) in which the parents of a child born with Tay-Sachs disease sought recovery for the trauma they endured witnessing their child succumbing to that degenerative disorder. The Court in both cases declined, for policy reasons, to sanction the recovery of damages for psychic or emotional harm occasioned by the birth and gradual death of a child.

The question as to whether the child has a cause of action for damages for "wrongful life" has mainly been decided in the negative, and damages have been considered as being too speculative despite an alleged breach of duty by the physician to the child. Therefore, and notwithstanding the birth of an afflicted child, damages to the child rather than to the parents will not be considered. This is of immense importance to a practitioner because of the statute of limitations problem. If the claim of "wrongful life" were recognized, the physician could face the responsibility many years after the fact, and even after 1975, in New York State, could face a claim made almost thirteen years after the claimed commission of the active negligence. The statute of limitations is considerably shorter when the parents are the claimant, since the statute is not tolled, as in the case of the minor; rather than a possible period of liability of almost thirteen years, the period can be less than three years.

The differences are of great importance. Although the infant cannot bring claim for being born, it can bring claim for damages based on negligence, and that claim is tolled by most statutes of limitations. Negligent administration of drugs causing damage to the infant could result in a claim against the physician, by the infant, many years later.

Physician Liability and Drugs

Research could easily provide a table or list of cases in which various acts have resulted in verdicts against or in favor of the physician. Such a compilation would not be helpful nor could it be relied upon to determine liability in the future. The use of a particular drug or of a particular medical procedure is subject to constant review and revision. Even the standard of care by which the physician's act is measured is not precise and changes frequently. As the knowledge of the medical community increases and as the standard of care in the community improves, a physician is held to an ever-increasing standard. The requirement that a physician keep abreast of his field and of the current state of the art becomes imperative from a liability standpoint.

Administration of Drugs

In New York State, a practitioner administering drugs to expectant mothers should be thoroughly familiar with Section 2503 of the Public Health Law of the State of New York. That Section provides:

The physician or nurse-midwife to be in attendance at the birth of a child shall inform the expectant mother, in advance of the birth, of the drugs that such physician or nurse-midwife expects to employ during pregnancy and of the obstetrical and other drugs that such physician or nurse-midwife expects to employ at birth and of the possible effects of such drugs on the child and mother.

Violation of Section 2503 of the Public Health Law of the State of New York, could be considered as medical malpractice. Although the section would, at first, appear to be an informed consent statute, it might not be so construed by the courts. If a violation of the statute were considered as negligence per se, it probably would not be necessary to call an expert physician witness, even in those instances which occur after July 1, 1975.

It is apparent that physicians administering drugs to expectant mothers which might have an effect on either the mother or the fetus, must not only be familiar with the current state of the art as to medical information concerning the drugs, but must also be familiar with the current law of the community in which they practice.

Since the ultimate question of liability is always decided by a jury of laymen, assisted but not bound by the advice of expert physicians, it is impossible to set forth a detailed codification of procedures which are acceptable and unacceptable. In the field of fetal medication, the effects of thalidomide and DES are too obvious to be used as examples. Other medications in which the effects are not yet clear are in a constant state of research, investigation and observation. By the time this book is published, the information available concerning drugs frequently used in prenatal care may have expanded considerably. The purpose of this chapter, therefore, is to advise the general principles upon which the standard of care will be applied. The rather narrow question of liability for the administration of drugs to a pregnant woman requires an analysis of the available knowledge of the effect of those drugs on the woman and on the fetus at the time they are administered. While there might not be a cause of action for "wrongful life," there is certainly a cause of action for "wrongful birth" which, although allowable only to the parents and having a rather short statute of limitations, must still be considered a potential liability.

The question of liability is an easy question at the extremes. The question of liability for the current prescription of thalidomide to a pregnant woman is obvious. It is also obvious that the administration of any drug which causes no harmful effect on the fetus or the mother can cause no liability. Unfortunately, most situations fall between the two obvious extremes.

It is evident the physician has the responsibility for choosing the appropriate drug and for monitoring its effects and side effects. The manufacturer is responsible for producing and marketing a drug free of contaminating organisms and materials, and for pre-marketing testing of the drug to determine its effectiveness and to prove its safety, and to advise the physician of the dangers and side effects of the drug.

The use of any particular drug must be in strict accordance with the information received; variations of the use for conditions not named in the official labeling caused the Food and Drug Administration to issue a drug bulletin in October, 1972, warning physicians of a malpractice potential for following unapproved practices. It goes without saying that patients receiving medication are to be warned against and monitored for any adverse effects. The warning need not be all-inclusive, but may only include a warning of the earlier signs and symptoms of a particular drug reaction. It might not necessarily include a description of catastrophic events which would occur only if the early signs were disregarded. In some cases, injury may be a consequence of the side effect rather than the side effect itself (such as in drugs producing drowsiness).

Under much discussion throughout the United States is the use of the "time of discovery" rule as opposed to the "first breath rule." The "time of discovery" rule would allow claims to be made within a period of time after the injury was discovered. The "first breath" rule would limit claims to the earliest possible date and require that they be brought within the appropriate statute of limitations thereafter. In New York State this argument was settled in 1979 by the Court of Appeals ruling in *Thornton v. Roosevelt Hospital* (47 N.Y.2d 780). In that decision the Court stated, "It is well established in this state that when chemical compounds are injected into a person's body, the injury occurs upon the drugs introduction not when the alleged deleterious effects of its component chemicals become apparent...We decline the invitation to extend judicially the discovery rule to strict liability action. Such matter is best reserved for the legislature and not the courts."

Prima Facie Tort

An additional recent development in New York State has been a decision from the state's highest court denying physicians the right to sue former patients who had previously unsuccessfully brought claims against the physician. The physicians' claims were based upon the theory of prima facie tort, which is a wrong occasioned by a lawful act done solely out of malice and ill will to injure another. In 1978 the court decided *Drago v. Buonagurio* (46 NY2d 778) and in 1979 the court decided *Belsky v. Lowenthal* (47 NY2d 820), both involving suits by physicians against former patients. The decisions in both cases severely narrowed the scope of the prima facie tort. In the Drago case, the physician alleged that he and others involved were sued in an action brought by a patient, by the patient's administrator, initiated at the direction of one of the defendants, an attorney. The complaint alleged that the decedent had never been the physician's patient, nor had the physician treated him directly or indirectly during the illness which allegedly caused his death, and that there was absolutely no basis for designating the physician as a defendant in the lawsuit. The physician claimed that it was done indiscriminately and only as a discovery device in order to secure evidence against the other defendant. The complaint also alleged that the attorney's actions in bringing the suit against the physician, were malicious, unethical and grossly negligent, and that the physician suffered mental anguish, injury to reputation and other damages. The Court of Appeals, in an unanimous decision decided that the physician's complaint failed to state a cause of action in either abusive process, malicious prosecution or negligence. The Court ruled that even if all of the allegations contained in the physician's complaint were true, they still did not justify legal action, and the case was dismissed. The Court of Appeals also refused to consider the claim of the physician based upon a claim of prima facie tort.

In the second matter decided by the Court of Appeals, *Belsky v. Lowenthal,* Mrs. Lowenthal, at the age of 30 years, decided to conceive and bear a child. Her husband, then 65 years of age, was opposed to their becoming parents. Mrs. Lowenthal became pregnant, which the plaintiff, as her physician, confirmed. She thereafter told her husband, falsely, that the plaintiff physician had stated that she was not pregnant. Knowing full well that she was pregnant, Mrs. Lowenthal delayed informing her husband until her pregnancy was so far advanced as to make an abortion—which she knew he would insist upon her having—medically dangerous to her health. She thereafter bore a son. Mrs. Lowenthal and her still deceived husband sued the physician for malpractice in the amount of $40,000,000. That action was later discontinued with prejudice, by stipulation. The physician then sued the Lowenthals, claiming in essence, that Mrs. Lowenthal had deliberately placed him in the position of being subjected to the lawsuit and that when the lawsuit was later discontinued against him, it was all part of a scheme by Mrs. Lowenthal to use the physician as an excuse for having gone against her husband's desires. The Court of Appeals, again in an unanimous decision, refused to recognize the physician's suit based upon a claim of prima facie tort. It also refused to recognize the cause of action in any of the traditional torts. Again, the highest court in the State of New York has left it to the legislature to correct an unconscionable decision, if in fact the result is unconscionable.

SUMMARY AND CONCLUSIONS

It is self-evident that medicine cannot be practiced without risks which include the possibility of malpractice claims. The physician can reduce those risks by keeping abreast of the available knowledge, practicing within the standards of the community, avoiding dealing in areas in which he or she is not fully qualified, obtaining informed consent, and maintaining a personal contact with the patient based on mutual trust and respect. These basic principles are also self-evident and are in any event, difficult for a dedicated professional to overlook.

BIBLIOGRAPHY

Buchsbaum, HJ: Trauma in Pregnancy, 1979.

Kaminetzky, HA and Iffy, L: Progress in Perinatology, 1977.

Liability for Failure of Birth Control Methods, 1976 Columbia Law Review 1187.

Wrongful Birth in the Abortion Context: Critique of existing case law and proposal for future actions, 1953 Denver Law Journal 501, 1976.

Wrongful Birth and Emotional Distress Damages: Suggested Approach, 1936 University of Pittsburgh Law Review 550, 1977.

The Impact of Medical Knowledge on the Law Relating to Prenatal Injuries, 110 University of Pennsylvania Law Review, 554, 1962.

The Unborn Child, University of Toronto Law Journal, 279, 1942.

The Unborn Plaintiff, 1963 Michigan Law Review 579, 1965.

Civil Liability for Prenatal Injuries, 40 Modern Law Review, 141, 1977.

Sins of the Fathers, Tort Liability for Prenatal Injuries, 90 Quarterly Law Review, 531, 1974.

Claim for Wrongful Conception, 24 Journal of Reproductive Medicine, 51, 1980.

Gleitman v. Cosgrove, 49 N.J.22,227 A.(2d) 689 (Supreme Court of New Jersey, 1967).

Custodio v. Bauer, 59 Cal. Rptr.463 (Court of Appeals, 1967).

Troppi v. Scarf, 31 Mich, App.240,187 N.W. (2d)511 (Court of Appeals, 1971).

Terrell v. Garcia, 496 S.W.(2d) 124 (Texas Court of Appeals, 1973).

Cox v. Stretton, 77 Misc.(2d)155,352 N.Y. Supp.(2d) 834 (Supreme Court).

Rieck v. Medical Protective Company of Fort Wayne, 64 Wisc.(2d)514,219 N.W.(2d) (Supreme Court of Wisconsin, 1974).

Ziemba v. Sternberg, 45 A.D.(2d)230,357 N.Y. Supp.(2d) 265 (Supreme Court of New York, Appellate Division, 1974).

Coleman v. Garrison, 327 A.(2d) 757 (Superior Court, New Castle, Delaware, 1974).

Betancourt v. Gaylor, 136 N.J. Super 69,344 A.(2d) 336 (Superior Court of New Jersey, 1975).

Anonymous v. State, 33 Conn. Sup.126,366 A.(2d) 204 (Superior Court of Connecticut, 1976).

Stills v. Gratton, 55 Cal. App.(3rd)698, 128 Cal Rptr. 652 (California Court of Appeals, First District, 1976).

Howard v. Lecher, 53 A.D.(2d) 420,386 N.Y. Supp.(2d)460 (Supreme Court of New York, Appellate Division 1976).

Bowman v. Davis, 48 Ohio St.(2d)41,2,Ohio Ops.(3d)41 (Supreme Court of Ohio, 1976).

Clegg v. Chase, 89 Misc.(2d)510,391 N.Y.Supp.(2d) 966 (Supreme Court of New York, Orange County, 1977).

Karlsons v. Guerinot, 57 A.D.(2d)73,394 N.Y.Supp. (2d)933 (New York Supreme Court. Fourth Appellate Division, 1977).

Sherlock v. Stillwater, 260 N.W.(2d) 169 (Supreme Court of Minnesota, 1977).

Park v. Chessin, 60 A.D.(2d)80 400 N.Y.Supp.(2d)110 (Supreme Court of New York, Second Appellate Division, 1977).

Becker v. Schwartz, 60A.D.(2d)587,400 N.Y.Supp.(2d) 119 (Supreme Court of New York, Second Appellate Division, 1977).

Green v. Sudakin, 81 Mich.App.545,265 N.W.(2d) 411 (Court of Appeals of Michigan, 1978).

Rivera v. State, 94 Misc.(2d)157,404 N.Y.Supp.(2d) 950 (Court of Claims of New York, 1978).

Mark DJ: Liability for failure of birth control methods. Columbia Law Rev 76:1187, 1976.

Veazey LH: An action for wrongful life brought on behalf of the wrongfully conceived infant. Wake Forest Law Rev. 13:712, 1977.

Marden, G Dixon, Drug Product Liability, 1977.

The Case of the Unwanted Blessing: Wrongful Life (31 U Miami L. Rev1409) Kashi.

Tedeschi, On Tort Liability for "Wrongful Life" (1 Israel L. Rev 513).

A Cause of Action for "Wrongful Life": (A Suggested Analysis) (55 Minn L. Rev 58).

Torts Prior to Conception: A New Theory of Liability (56 Neb L. Rev 706).

Remedy for the Reluctant Parent: Physicians' Liability for the Post-Sterilization, Conception and Birth of Unplanned Children (27 U Fla L. Rev 158).

Father and Mother Know Best: Defining the Liability of Physicians for Inadequate Genetic Counseling (87 Yale LJ 1488).

Strict Liability: A "Lady in Waiting" for Wrongful Birth Cases (11 Cal W L Rev 136).

146

Wrongful Birth: The Emerging Status of a New Tort (8 St. Mary's LJ 140).

Preconception Torts: Foreseeing the Unconceived (48 U Col L Rev 621).

Morris, Wrongful Birth in the Abortion Context, (53 Denver LJ 501).

Sexual Sterilization, (21 Am Jur) Proof of Facts 255.

N. Y. Civil Practice Law and Rules, Section 214; (Statute of Limitations).

N. Y. Civil Practice Law and Rules, Section 208, (Statute of Limitations).

N. Y. Civil Practice Law and Rules, Section 4401; (Informed Consent Requiring Expert Testimony).

31 Syracuse Law Review 1 "1979 Survey of New York Law".

N.Y. Pattern Jury Instructions, 2nd Edition, 1974.

Plante, An Analysis of Informed Consent, 36 Fordham Law Review 639.

Coffey, Assault on Informed Consent, 48 N.Y.S.Bar Jur. 447.

Marks, Informed Consent in Medical Malpractice Cases, 17. For the Defense.

Gair, Informed Consent of Patient as a Pre-requisite to Medical and Surgical Treatment, 2 University of West Los Angeles Law Review, 61.

45 C.F.R. Sec. 46.109(1976)

45 C.F.R. Sec. 46.103(c)(1976)

46 C.F.R. Sec. 46.109 (1976)

Schneyer, Informed Consent and the Danger of Bias in the Formation of Medical Disclosure Practices, 1976, Wis. L. Rev. 124.

Waltz and Scheuneman, Informed Consent to Therapy, 1970, 64 Nw. U.L. Rev. 628.

Index

Numerals in *italics* indicate a figure, "t" indicates tabular matter.